My First nMRCGP Book

Also available from Remedica
My First MRCP Book Second Edition

Published by Remedica
Commonwealth House, 1 New Oxford Street, London, WC1A 1NU, UK
Sears Tower, 233 South Wacker Drive, Suite 3425, IL 60606, USA

books@remedica.com
www.remedica.com
Tel: +44 (0)20 7759 2999
Fax: +44 (0)20 7759 2951

Publisher: Andrew Ward
In-house editors: Catherine Booth and Naomi McCormick
Design and Artwork: AS&K Skylight Creative Services

ISBN: 978-1-901346-86-2
British Library Cataloguing-in-Publication Data.
A catalogue record for this book is available from the British Library.

Printed in Malta

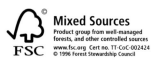

My First nMRCGP Book

Penny Moore
Summertown Health Centre
Oxford, UK

Simon Curtis
19 Beaumont Street Surgery
Oxford, UK

REMEDICA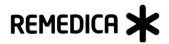

To our fathers, Adam Locket and Robert Curtis,
both wonderful teachers and inspirations.

Acknowledgements

We would like to thank:

Dr Carl Heneghan, who wrote the evidence-based medicine section of an earlier draft of this book designed for the 'old' MRCGP examination. Although this section then had to be dropped due to the shift in emphasis in the new exam, we are very grateful for his hard work and input, and heartily recommend the excellent book *Evidence-Based Medicine Toolkit* by Heneghan and Badenoch to all as recompense!

Andrew Moore for wise advice and encouragement; the adorable Cathy Curtis for her careful reading of the text, suggested comments and changes and her infinite patience at the piles of boring books and papers cluttering up the house.

The many GP registrars we have had contact with over the years, both at the Oxford District Vocational Training Scheme and at NB Medical Education's Hot Topics courses. Their input on the issues that matter to them, and first hand experience of the nMRCGP examination, has been invaluable in putting this book together.

Our excellent editor Naomi McCormick for her encouraging and professional guidance.

Our colleagues in our practices and at the Oxford Deanery for their encouragement, and in particular Jill Edwards.

Richard Stevens, for encouraging Penny to think outside boxes.

Numerous books, journals and websites have been ploughed through to research this book. There are too many to acknowledge, but the two that stand out as essential founts of information are: the official RCGP website for its very detailed and comprehensive guidance to the new curriculum and exam, and *The Condensed Curriculum Guide* by Riley, Haynes and Field.

Penny Moore and Simon Curtis

About the authors

Penny Moore is a GP partner and trainer at Summertown Health Centre, Oxford, and a programme director for the Oxford District GP Vocational Training Scheme. She did her undergraduate training in Australia and her GP training in Oxford. She previously lectured for NB Medical Education's Hot Topics course.

Simon Curtis is a GP and medical educator. He is a GP partner at 19 Beaumont Street, a training practice in central Oxford, and has previously practised in Australia and Italy. He is the co-founder of NB Medical Education's Hot Topics course and also has experience as a Vocational Training Scheme course organiser.

Contents

Introduction   VIII

Glossary   X

1. How and why?   1

2. The applied knowledge test   15

3. Clinical skills assessment   35

4. Workplace-based assessment   57

Appendix 1:   My first guide to evidence-based
                medicine and critical appraisal   87

Appendix 2:   Ethics, mental capacity and
                values-based practice   99

Appendix 3:   Consultation models   103

Appendix 4:   Consultation observation tool
                marking schedule   109

Index   113

Introduction

We may be biased, but we believe that general practice is both the best and the hardest job in medicine. GPs must juggle multiple clinical problems, deal with worried relatives, eccentric colleagues and positively bizarre government directives, and stay up to date with the latest treatments, all of the while consulting at 10-minute intervals and maintaining their sense of humour.

In return, the job is never boring or predictable, and when you do it well you not only gain real clinical satisfaction, but also the trust and respect of your patients and the community. While our hospital colleagues are specialising themselves into corners, we remain broad in outlook – genuinely skilled, caring GPs. What a great job!

There's only one catch. Before you can become a GP you must clear the hurdle of the nMRCGP examination, which has become compulsory and is based on the most enormously complicated curriculum. The curriculum runs to hundreds of pages, and if printed out (do **not** try this at home) would use more paper than a large-print version of *War and Peace*. To make it even more complicated, the RCGP divides the curriculum up into *domains*, *competencies*, *competences* and *disciplines*, as well as the more usual *skills*, *attitudes* and *knowledge*. It also 'maps' in strange and mysterious ways. The examination itself, with its many acronyms and subacronyms and tests within tests, can also seem unfathomable.

But the good news is this: **ultimately, the RCGP is looking for sensible, broad-thinking, caring, holistic doctors who can use, integrate and apply what they know**. That's what the curriculum and the examination boil down to – honest!

This book will help you to learn the essential skills of general practice and pass the nMRCGP examination. It is what it says on the cover: your *First nMRCGP Book*, in that it will give you a brief introduction and a way into the rather complicated new world of GP training and assessment. This is not an official guide, but we (the authors) have years of experience in teaching, training and assessing GPs within the NHS. Our experience has taught us that starting with a clear basic outline and keeping the big picture in view are the keys to success.

We recommend that you progress from this book to the other, more detailed publications that are available, but that you remember our mantra: **the nMRCGP examination is straightforward, as long as you can see the wood for the trees.**

Our aim in writing this book is to help you keep a clear mind, assist you with structuring your learning, enthuse you and maybe raise a few smiles along the way. We hope it will bring pleasure and clarity, and that any readers with a more serious disposition will forgive our analogies and humour. General practice is a serious business, but being a GP should be fun.

How to use this book

This book has been designed to complement the many resources and tools that are available on the RCGP's website (www.rcgp.org.uk), as well as the many other excellent knowledge bases and textbooks that are available, which we strongly encourage you to buy and use.

We will keep bringing you back to basics, common sense and the bottom line, because these are what you need not just to pass the examination, but also to be a good GP. This approach has always helped to keep us relatively sane, and that is what we hope to pass on to you.

- **Chapter 1**, *How and Why*, deals with the overall structure of the examination and what it is testing.

- **Chapters 2**, **3** and **4** deal with the three main parts of the examination: the *Applied Knowledge Test*, *Clinical Skills Assessment* and *Workplace-Based Assessment*.

- More detailed and referenced information regarding ethics, evidence-based practice and other key areas are included as **Appendices**.

We've actually employed some educational theory here, to do with right- and left-brain learning and so on. Learning should be pleasurable and should make you feel positive, so, most importantly, when using this book on your way to becoming a (**n**ew) **M**agnificent and **R**eally **C**ool **GP**... HAVE FUN!

Glossary

Acronymitis: the play

[Two people, one young, bright and attractive (GPR – think yourself) the other middle-aged, grey and sallow (GPT – think Bill Nighy) are in the CR having a T.]

GPT: OK, let's do a CBD. We'll look at the COT, but first, how did it go with Mrs Smith?

GPR: Well, I think. Her PEFRs are better. Oh, and I ticked all of the QOF boxes on EMIS.

GPT: Uhmm…, OK. PEFRs are PDI for the nMRCGP examination, and we'll do DOPS for the WPBA and CSA. It's also important for the RITA and QOF, but maybe for Mrs Smith we should be more interested in POO?

GPR: POO? But she came for an asthma check…

GPT: You're right. OK, OK… PEFRs are important DOOs for CDM, EBM, the NICE/SIGN guidelines, CG and the QOF, but if we don't look at POO what will she think? What would she say in a PSQ? Maybe we need 360-degree MSF on this.

GPR: I'm sorry, I've no idea what you're on about…

GPT: Don't worry. That's because I'm WAC and you're YAN. *[GPT leans forward, smiling.]* Look, let's KISS.

GPR: KISS?!!

GPT: OK, OK, relax… If you don't want to KISS, let's do a CEX instead. *[GPR presses panic button.]*

If you, too, suffer from nMRCGP examination acronymitis (symptoms include brain ache, anger, irrational laughter and total bewilderment) and feel lost in its Kafkaesque world then we hope that the following 'prescription' may help.

Acronymitis: the prescription

AiT associate in training

That's you. PDQ after your AKT, CSA and WPBA you'll be an AiT GPStR nMRCGP. Wow!

AKT applied knowledge test

The MCQ component of the nMRCGP examination.

CBD case-based discussion

Used to be called a "chat about Mrs Smith", now a structured WPBA tool.

CDM chronic disease management

CEX clinical evaluation exercise

I know. You couldn't make it up. The only thing worse is mini-CEX, a WPBA tool.

CG clinical governance

COT consultation observation tool

This used to be a video camera but now it's a structured form for assessing recorded consultations: a WPBA tool.

CPD continuing professional development

CR consulting room

CrAp critical appraisal

CSA clinical skills assessment

The 'OSCE where you consult with struggling actors' component of the nMRCGP examination.

CSR clinical supervisor's report

Like the dreaded school report discussed at parents' evening. Used for hospital placements as a WPBA tool.

DENS doctors' educational needs

DOE disease-orientated evidence

Similar to DOO, below.

DOO   disease-orientated outcome
                   As opposed to POO.

DOPS   direct observation of procedural skills
                   This acronym with rhythm used to be called "You have a go and I'll watch,"
                   another recorded WPBA tool. Fortunately, a PR and prostate examination can
                   be included in the same DOPS…

EMQ   extended matching question
                   A question type in the AKT.

GPR   general practice registrar

GPT   general practice trainer

GSOH   good sense of humour
                   Absolutely essential!

IM&T   information management and technology
                   IT just got more complicated.

KISS   keep it simple, stupid

MBA   multiple best answer

MCQ   multiple choice question

MSF   multisource feedback
                   This is another WPBA tool. Best be nice to all of your colleagues. Don't get paranoid.

NICE   National Institute for Health and Clinical Excellence

nMRCGP   new Membership of the Royal College of General Practitioners examination
examination

OSCE   Objective Structured Clinical Examination
                   The model for the CSA.

PDI   pretty damn interesting

PDP   personal development plan

PDQ	pretty damn quick
PEFR	peak expiratory flow rate
PMETB	Postgraduate Medical Education and Training Board
	The regulatory body that oversees GP training and approves the curriculum and the nMRCGP examination. Therefore also known as 'the scapegoat'.
POEM	patient-orientated evidence that matters
	A research paper that looks at PEFR would be DOE, whilst one that assesses the symptoms of breathlessness is POEM.
POO	patient-orientated outcome
	As an example, in asthma a PEFR is a DOO, but breathlessness is a POO.
PSQ	patient satisfaction questionnaire
	Best be nice to your patients as well because this is a WPBA tool. You'll just have to take it out on the cat.
PSR	pet satisfaction report
	There's no escape.
PUNS	patients' unmet needs
	A popular way of identifying learning needs by noting which of a patient's information 'needs' you were unable to meet.
QOF	quality and outcomes framework of the GP contract
RITA	record of in-training assessment
	Educating Rita *was way ahead of its time.*
SBA	single best answer
	The most common question type in the AKT.
T	tutorial
TAC	table/algorithm completion
	The rarest question type in the AKT. You 'fill in the gaps'.
TLC	tender loving care

WAC   wise and clever

WPBA   workplace-based assessment

This is the continual assessment component of the nMRCGP examination and is based, er, in the workplace. It uses MSF, PSQ, COT, CBD, DOPS, mini-CEX and CSR as tools to gather evidence of competence.

YAN   young and naïve

1. How & why?

Overview of the nMRCGP and the curriculum: seeing the wood for the trees

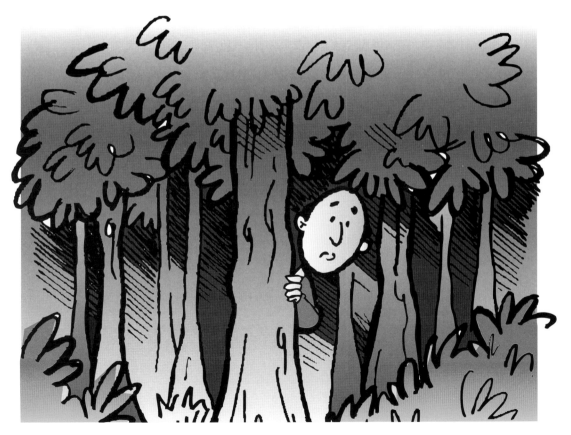

Before we start, we want you to repeat after us:
**The nMRCGP examination is straightforward,
as long as you can see the wood for the trees.**

This statement is our key message.

Read it, learn it and repeat it.

Write it on your bathroom door.

Believe it.

You will be able to find hundreds of pages on the RCGP website about the various parts of the examination, the curriculum and so on. There are also some great books coming out. While the detail is important, we think that it is hard to get an overview, so here is ours.

First, the ultrasimplistic simplification

- There is a new examination.
- The examination is based on a new syllabus (which is about what can be tested).
- The syllabus is based on a new curriculum (which describes what a good GP should know and be).
- The curriculum is based on the General Medical Council's (GMC's) guidance, *Good Medical Practice*.

Why was it changed?

Previously, Summative Assessment (an assessment of minimal competence) and the MRCGP examination (an assessment of excellence) sat side by side in a confused sort of way, resulting in duplication of assessment, frazzled registrars, and a membership qualification, which, unlike those of other specialties, was not an essential requirement for practising as a GP. The public wanted reassurance that their GPs were safe, competent and caring. The advent of the Postgraduate Medical Education and Training Board (PMETB) and the *Mangling*, oops, *Modernising Medical Careers* programme demanded a proper curriculum, so someone had to write one down and devise a way of assessing it.

If you like, at this stage you can visit the RCGP's website or your e-portfolio and see how the nMRCGP examination 'maps' across the curriculum. Alternatively, you could have a chocolate biscuit and resume reading below. (Later on, the mapping is a useful tool to guide you in your learning, but early in your training it can give you brain overload.)

How does the nMRCGP examination fit in with general practice and 'real life'?

The nMRCGP examination is designed to be more relevant to real life than the old MRCGP examination. As such, it includes an assessment of you as an apprentice-in-practice as you hone your skills. **Seeing the wood for the trees** is essential, because the ability to see through to the heart of the matter, be it in diagnosis, dealing with a difficult patient or negotiating with your partnership, is what makes a truly good GP. At least some of the assessment process looks for this. The nMRCGP examination is also about being a Good Doctor, as defined by the GMC (see 'Good Medical Practice' later in this chapter). We will tell you more about the examination later, don't worry.

Where does the curriculum come from?

Good Medical Practice

The GP curriculum and the nMRCGP syllabus dovetail with the essential GMC document *Good Medical Practice*, which is very reassuring! To remind you, here are: a) the statement *The Duties of a Doctor Registered with the General Medical Council*, and b) the contents of *Good Medical Practice*.

The Duties of a Doctor Registered with the General Medical Council[a]

Patients must be able to trust doctors with their lives and health. To justify that trust you must show respect for human life and you must:

- make the care of your patient your first concern
- protect and promote the health of patients and the public
- provide a good standard of practice and care
  - keep your professional knowledge and skills up to date
  - recognise and work within the limits of your competence
  - work with colleagues in the ways that best serve patients' interests
- treat patients as individuals and respect their dignity
  - treat patients politely and considerately
  - respect patients' right to confidentiality
- work in partnership with patients
  - listen to patients and respond to their concerns and preferences
  - give patients the information they want or need in a way they can understand
  - respect patients' right to reach decisions with you about their treatment and care
  - support patients in caring for themselves to improve and maintain their health
- be honest and open and act with integrity
  - act without delay if you have a good reason to believe that you or a colleague may be putting patients at risk
  - never discriminate unfairly against patients or colleagues
  - never abuse your patients' trust in you or the public's trust in the profession

You are personally accountable for your professional practice and must always be prepared to justify your decisions and actions.

---

[a]From *Good Medical Practice*, General Medical Council, 2006.

The contents of *Good Medical Practice*

Good clinical care

Providing good clinical care

Supporting self-care

Avoid treating those close to you

Raising concerns about patient safety

Decisions about access to medical care

Treatment in emergencies

Maintaining good medical practice

Keeping up to date

Maintaining and improving your performance

Teaching and training, appraising and assessing

Relationships with patients

The doctor–patient partnership

Good communication

Children and young people

Relatives, carers and partners

Being open and honest with patients if things go wrong

Maintaining trust in the profession

Consent

Confidentiality

Ending your professional relationship with a patient

Working with colleagues

Working in teams

Conduct and performance of colleagues

Respect for colleagues

Arranging cover

Taking up and ending appointments

Sharing information with colleagues

Delegation and referral

Probity

Being honest and trustworthy

Publishing and providing information about your services

Writing reports and CVs, giving evidence and signing documents

Research

Financial and commercial dealings

Conflicts of interest

Health (your own)

Good Medical Practice is the blueprint of blueprints. We suggest that you read it often to remind you where the heart of the curriculum lies, and where your heart should lie.

> "Patients need good doctors. Good doctors make the care of their patients their first concern: they are competent, keep their knowledge and skills up to date, establish and maintain good relationships with patients and colleagues, are honest and trustworthy, and act with integrity."
>
> ***Good Medical Practice***, General Medical Council, 2006

Coping with the curriculum

Although it is great to have a proper curriculum at last to define and focus learning, it is clear that it was written by several different committees. It's huge, repetitive and frankly quite hard to understand at times. So, where do you begin and how on earth do you cope? We will help you to make a start and to continue in a sane, uncomplicated way, as follows...

First, a desensitising exercise

Take a deep breath, relax and look at the curriculum contents (see page 6). That wasn't too bad, was it? Now try it again, repeating the statement, **the nMRCGP examination is straightforward, as long as you can see the wood for the trees.**

A few tips

- Do **not** attempt to download and print the whole curriculum – your printer will explode and so will your brain.

- Remember: the curriculum is a tool to help you, not a stick to beat yourself with.

- Think of it as a useful map, designed to lead to interesting places. It can show you the possibilities, but you need to accept that you'll never reach all of them.

- Read the GMC document *Good Medical Practice*.

- Read (or if your practice doesn't have a copy, buy) *The Condensed Curriculum Guide* (see 'Resources', later in this chapter) and start using it. It summarises the curriculum areas and provides lots of useful references and resources.

- Log onto the e-portfolio (see **Chapter 4**) and start cruising around the various templates, tick-boxes and links. When you start to feel sick, log out and do something else.

- Read the core statement of the curriculum, *Being a General Practitioner*.

- Make use of the resources listed on the RCGP's website (www.rcgp.org.uk).

Now go back to your new mantra: **the nMRCGP examination is straightforward, as long as you can see the wood for the trees.** As you can see from the curriculum contents, straightforward clinical management areas come after the bigger, broader stuff. This is not an accident, but reflects the emphasis on the very special skills and attitudes that are needed to be a good GP.

The contents of the RCGP curriculum for general practice

1. Core statement – being a general practitioner
2. The general practice consultation
3. Personal and professional responsibilities
   3.1. Clinical governance
   3.2. Patient safety
   3.3. Clinical ethics and values-based practice
   3.4. Promoting equality and valuing diversity
   3.5. Evidence-based practice
   3.6. Research and academic activity
   3.7. Teaching, mentoring and clinical supervision
4. Management
   4.1. Management in primary care
   4.2. Information management and technology
5. Healthy people: promoting health and preventing disease
6. Genetics in primary care
7. Care of acutely ill people
8. Care of children and young people
9. Care of older adults
10. Gender-specific health issues
    10.1. Women's health
    10.2. Men's health
11. Sexual health
12. Care of people with cancer and palliative care
13. Care of people with mental health problems
14. Care of people with learning disabilities
15. Clinical management
    15.1. Cardiovascular problems
    15.2. Digestive problems
    15.3. Drug and alcohol problems
    15.4. Ear, nose and throat and facial problems
    15.5. Eye problems
    15.6. Metabolic problems
    15.7. Neurological problems
    15.8. Respiratory problems
    15.9. Rheumatology and conditions of the musculoskeletal system (including trauma)
    15.10. Skin problems

The core statement

We aren't going to spend much more time on the curriculum, except for this bit. The RCGP considers *The Core Statement – Being a General Practitioner* to be of vital importance. It breaks down the main areas of the curriculum into 10 'domains'.

- six core competences (broad areas of expertise)

- three essential application features of the discipline of general practice (features that influence how you use the core competences)

- psychomotor skills (specific practical and clinical skills)

We think that these areas need demystifying so we've given our interpretation of each below. They are actually all about common sense and explain where the examination is coming from. They also show why GPs are special. **Don't** get hung up on them. **Do** bear in mind the breadth of general practice, and that what you need to learn is so much more than facts. This is how general practice (and the nMRCGP examination) is so different from other disciplines, and why it's such a great job.

The six core competences

1. Primary care management

GPs deal with patients at the coalface. Patients may present with any problem, in any order, with any background. You should know how to work with your own team and with other teams, and know when and how to refer. You should also be able to juggle demands, needs and resources. Be an advocate for the patient. Easy.

2. Person-centred care

This is about listening to the patient, finding out why they came and working in partnership with them to reach a solution. Piece of cake. (There is more on this in **Chapter 4**.)

3. Specific problem-solving skills

These are skills that every doctor needs: decision making, clinical reasoning and management of emergencies – but with big differences from our hospital colleagues. You know the old joke about hearing horses' hooves in the distance, and the hospital physician saying: "Aha! I hear a unicorn!" Marshall Marinker famously differentiated hospital doctors from GPs like this:

- Hospital doctors have to reduce uncertainty, explore possibility and marginalize error ("Could be a unicorn, better organise a serum hoof count and PET scan, just in case it is a unicorn and it scratches us with its nasty sharp pointy horn").

- Whilst GPs must tolerate uncertainty, explore probability and marginalize danger ("It's most likely a horse, there are lots of horses around at the moment and I recognise that hoof beat. Most horses go away by themselves. If it's a unicorn, we'll find out soon enough and then deal with it... those expensive tests would use valuable resources and aren't needed yet.")

4. A comprehensive approach

GPs must accept and cope with the fact that patients have lots of things wrong with them at once and lots of different needs, and that these needs change over time.

They must also adjust their focus to any or all of:

- health promotion – helping Humpty Dumpty lose a little bit of weight ("He eats like a sparrow, doctor") so that he can stay balanced on his wall

- prevention – stop Humpty falling off his wall, or perhaps provide padding or a mattress in the impact zone

- cure – help put him back together again

- care – hold his hand a bit

- rehabilitation – help him to get back on the wall and stay there

- palliation – poor Humpty can't be put back together again and needs some TLC

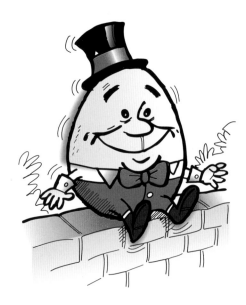

(And, of course, teamwork – all of the time working with All The King's Horses and All The King's Men.)

5. Community orientation

The health needs and resources of a seaside retirement town differ from those of an inner-city estate with a recent influx of refugees. As a GP, your work will be affected by these different needs and resources. Factors such as unemployment, ethnicity and housing will influence health and consulting behaviour. Commissioning, rationing and local healthcare systems all have to be understood and worked with. Of course, you know this already!

6. A holistic approach

Sadly, many hospital doctors still treat patients as if the only relevant factor is their disease, or as if they are a disease (eg, a pain in the backside). In contrast, good GPs understand their patients as complex 'whole' people, taking into account the following aspects:

- Psychological – "This pain in my bottom gets worse when I'm stressed."

- Social – "This pain in my bottom is making it really difficult to sit at my desk at work."

- Cultural – "I was always taught never to mention bottoms."

- Racial – "It is offensive to mention a female's bottom to a male in my culture."

- Religious beliefs – "In my religious sect, a pain in the bottom is a shameful thing."

- Expectations – "I expect the doctor will examine my bottom, which will be embarrassing, but if he doesn't then that wouldn't be thorough."

- Past experiences – "Uncle Joe had a pain like this in his bottom and it was cancer."

- Health beliefs – "It might be that blood pressure tablet causing it."

So far, so good. Remember:

The nMRCGP examination is straightforward, as long as you can see the wood for the trees.

The three essential application features of the discipline of general practice

These are three aspects of your personality and circumstances that influence how you put the competences into practise.

1. Contextual

This involves an awareness of the particular constraints and conditions under which GPs work. These differ from practice to practice.

2. Attitudinal

The effect of your own attitudes on how you look after your patients. This means awareness of your own limits, ethics, values and feelings, and of your work–life balance.

3. Scientific

Knowing the science of medicine, keeping up to date and knowing how to read and critically appraise research. In this context, being a swot is a Good Thing.

Psychomotor skills

No, not how to drive like the presenters on *Top Gear*. Sitting your applied knowledge test (AKT) at a Pearson VUE driving-test centre is as near as you get to that one… This refers to practical skills such as using an ophthalmoscope, taking a smear, assessing blood pressure and so on (see **Chapters 3** and **4**).

So that is how the RCGP divides up the curriculum, to describe what being a GP is. Wait, there's more…

The 12 nMRCGP competency areas

For some unfathomable reason the RCGP then produces 12 'nMRCGP competency areas', against which you are assessed in the various modules of the examination. You can map your progress against the competences in your e-portfolio.

Clear? We thought so. You may need to repeat your mantra now…

In order to keep the wood in view amongst the trees, we're not going to go into the competency areas in any more detail just now. But in fact, we have briefly touched on all of these topics already. You will find them in your e-portfolio as you start to log your progress. Here they are as headings only.

The 12 nMRCGP competency areas for assessment

1. Communication and consulting skills
2. Practising holistically
3. Data gathering and interpretation
4. Making a diagnosis/making decisions
5. Clinical management
6. Managing complexity and promoting health
7. Primary care administration and information management and technology
8. Working with colleagues and in teams
9. Community orientation
10. Maintaining performance, learning and teaching
11. Maintaining an ethical approach to practice
12. Fitness to practice

Exercise

The many faces of a GP

Another way to think about the curriculum is to list the various roles that a doctor might adopt in the course of ordinary practice.

Look at this picture and then think of a recent working day, especially if you are currently based in general practice. You probably functioned in at least 10 of these roles. So the lists that the RCGP has come up with are not that mystifying really, they're just stating the obvious: that GPs are brilliant and versatile quick-change artists. And as you know, being a GP requires immense skill and charisma, which you have in spades.

We've included a few roles that the RCGP doesn't list, but which we know to be true from our own experience.

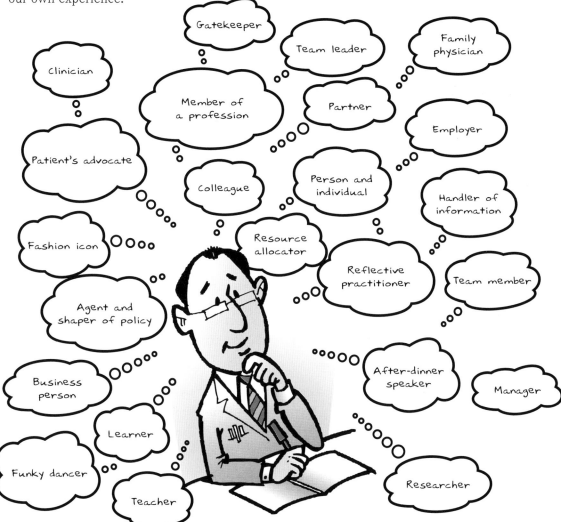

How does the nMRCGP examination work?

Membership by module

The nMRCGP is a membership-by-module examination. It's all quite familiar. Some sections of these modules resemble other specialty membership examinations, and others resemble assessments that you will have already encountered in hospital posts. Each of the three modules counts for an equal third of the total assessment.

- The AKT, which replaces the previous multiple choice question (MCQ) module, asks: do you know anything?

- The clinical skills assessment (CSA), which replaces the previous video module, asks: can you use, apply and integrate what you know when you see patients?

- The workplace-based assessment (WPBA), which is the really new bit, asks: are you a reasonable, sensible, broad-based, ethical team worker who can use, apply and integrate what you know, with real patients, in a real practice, alongside a real team, in a community? (Would you fulfil the 'maternity test'? That is: would my mum want you as her GP?)

Each of these modules is looked at in more detail in **Chapters 2**, **3** and **4**. You can resit the AKT and the CSA (see exam regulations on www.rcgp.org.uk). The WPBA must be completed by the end of your ST3 GP clinical attachment.

Key statements

Here are some key statements from the RCGP website about the nMRCGP examination and what we think they mean:

"It is derived from a blueprint using the specified knowledge, skills, behaviours and attitudes defined by the PMETB-approved RCGP training curriculum."

It's not just about what you know, but also about what you can do, and how you can apply and integrate your knowledge.

"It relates to the entire training period."

You begin the assessment process (particularly the WPBA) when you start your 3-year specialty training for general practice. Along the way, the numerous small assessments accumulate, building up a picture of your abilities in every area of general practice. Your progress is logged on your e-portfolio. External assessments (CSA and AKT) are intended to be sat in the final year of training.

"It is set at a standard expected of doctors being licensed to practise independently as general medical practitioners in the United Kingdom."

There is now one examination that will, at least in parts, be harder than the old Summative Assessment examination. What's good about the new format is that it looks at you in real life, in real practice, over time, as well as testing your knowledge and consulting skills more formally. There has, however, been much debate about whether the standard of the MRCGP will drop. Previously, there was much debate about whether the 'old' MRCGP adequately equipped people to be good GPs. As from now, none of that matters. What is important is that you are doing your membership examination, and you need to pass it.

How to enjoy your training while doing the nMRCGP

Some top tips from our experts:

- Be positive and optimistic – you are learning how to do a job that makes a real difference, and are on the threshold of a fantastic career.

- Keep looking for the wood amongst the trees.

- Start early and take control, don't procrastinate.

- Share your learning and experiences with others – join a study group, and turn up to learning sets and day-release education that has been arranged for you.

- Always have a good supply of chocolate.

- Be proactive about getting assessed and supervised (see **Chapter 4** on WPBA). Make contact with your clinical and educational supervisors early in your clinical attachments, and ensure that you get your various assessments done in plenty of time.

- 'Chunk' your knowledge learning into manageable pieces – 'eat the elephant slowly.'

- Work out how you learn best (eg, doing, reflecting, theorising, on your own or with groups) and initially arrange your learning to reflect your preferences. For instance, if you have a short attention span, do MCQs and learn piecemeal rather than trying to read long books from start to finish. However, you will have to branch out into other learning styles as you go on.

- Get into the habit of recording learning as it happens to you (see **Chapter 4**).

- Keep fit, healthy and happy outside of work.

- Remember that the examination is all about being (and showing that you are) a good doctor, which is what you want to be! Thankfully, if you keep this aim in mind, you will be on course for passing the nMRCGP examination.

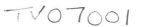

The following chapters will look in more detail at each module of the nMRCGP examination. As you go through these, remember: **the nMRCGP examination is straightforward, as long as you can see the wood for the trees.**

PATIENT: Doctor, I've swallowed a pillow!

DOCTOR: How do you feel?

PATIENT: A little down in the mouth...

Resources

Riley B, Haynes J, Field S. *The Condensed Curriculum Guide: for GP training and the new MRCGP.* London: Royal College of General Practitioners, 2007.

Royal College of General Practitioners. *Curriculum for Specialty Training for General Practice. The Core Statement: Being a General Practitioner.* London: Royal College of General Practitioners, 2007.

General Medical Council. *Good Medical Practice.* London: General Medical Council, 2006.

The Royal College of General Practitioners website: www.rcgp.org.uk.

2. The applied knowledge test

The **AKT** is enjoyable to prepare for and easy to pass

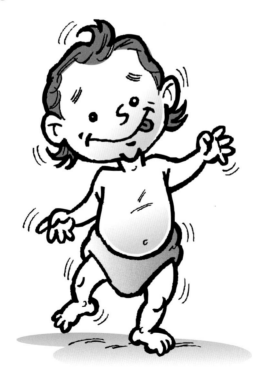

*"For a human being nothing comes naturally…
we have to learn everything we do."*
The Amber Spyglass, Philip Pullman

Compared with the mind-boggling acronyms and the crazy labyrinthine worlds of the workplace-based assessment (WPBA) and clinical skills assessment (CSA), the applied knowledge test (AKT) is beautifully and refreshingly simple. It may now be called an AKT and taken on a computer, but it remains a good old-fashioned multiple choice question (MCQ) examination. Remember the mantra: **the nMRCGP examination is straightforward, as long as you can see the wood for the trees.** To illustrate this, remember the famous story of the GP registrar and the trainer.

A GP trainer took his registrar camping on an induction weekend. In the middle of the night he woke up and shook his trainer awake:

GPR: Trainer, what do you see?

TRAINER: Why, I see a beautiful starry night.

GPR: So, what does that tell you?

TRAINER: [*Very pleased to be able to show off his knowledge.*] Well, astronomically speaking, I can see each of those stars is like our very own sun, releasing continuous energy by the nuclear fusion of hydrogen to helium. Astrologically, I can tell Pisces is about to enter Taurus, a very favourable time to take the AKT. Meteorologically speaking I see it's going to be a fine day tomorrow with some light showers in the early afternoon and horologically I can tell it's about 2.30 am. [*Then the trainer remembers he is supposed to reflect these questions back.*] But what does it tell you?

GPR: Well, it tells me that some bastard has nicked our tent.

Remember: **the nMRCGP examination is straightforward, as long as you can see the wood for the trees!**

This chapter is divided into:

- an overview of the AKT, including the good, the bad and the ugly

- the logistics: how to apply, what to expect and just who is Pearson VUE?

- preparation for the clinical aspects: umm, so how do I revise all of medicine?

- preparation for the nonclinical aspects: how can I tell an NNT from an FM3?

- question formats: what is the difference between a single best answer, extended matching question and table/algorithm completion?

- examination tips: how can I maximise my mark on the day?

Overview of the AKT: the good, the bad and the ugly

The good

If you are interested in clinical medicine, patients and the problems they present to GPs (and we daringly suggest that if you aren't you might be in the wrong job) then this is an examination that is enjoyable to prepare for and easy to pass. We repeat: enjoyable to prepare for, easy to pass. It has an instantly familiar format and is less challenging than the 'old' MRCGP MCQ examination. Furthermore, you will continue to use the tools and techniques that you develop in preparing for this examination throughout your career, eg, identifying learning needs and answering clinical queries using quality evidence sources.

The AKT really does test what you need to know in order to be a good GP. The RCGP define this as the knowledge that "underpins independent general practice in the UK in the context of the NHS". The distribution of the content is fair (medicine 80%, administration and management 10%, critical appraisal [CrAp] and evidence-based medicine [EBM] 10%) and the questions are directly relevant to your work, with the emphasis overwhelmingly on clinical scenarios.

The examination does what it says on the tin. It is testing how you can **apply** your **knowledge** in general practice. It is testing your clinical competence and problem-solving skills rather than your ability to recall facts. The topics are chosen on the basis that an 'ordinary GP' would be expected to have a working knowledge of them. It is crucial to remember this as you prepare.

Other plus points are:

- There is no negative marking! If you don't definitely know the answer, you can risk going on a hunch.

- There is plenty of time: 180 minutes for 200 items does not sound like much, but most people will find it more than enough.

- You no longer have to know loads of CrAp and the calculations are so simple that you don't need to bother with a calculator.

- The pass rate is high (in January 2008 the ST3 first-time pass rate was 88% [www.rcgp.org.uk]).

Essentially, the AKT is a game: a medical version of *Who Wants To Be a Millionaire?* or *Trivial Pursuit* and, like all games, it's fun as long as you know the rules and you're in the right frame of mind.

The bad

The level of question difficulty can be annoyingly inconsistent. Some questions may seem dumbed-down and simple, whilst others are esoteric. For each question there will be several correct responses, but which is the 'single best answer' can at times seem maddeningly subjective. Despite its familiar format, this module can be the most difficult to prepare for. How can you revise 'the whole of medicine'? In our experience, excellent candidates can slip up in the AKT. Our guide to preparation and examination tips will help to prevent this happening to you. There's no phone-a-friend (but it can be fun to think who you'd choose to phone if you could. Hands up who'd choose their trainer? No, thought not.), no 50:50 and, sadly, you can't ask the audience. In fact, they're so strict about this last bit that you can't even ask the person sitting next to you.

The ugly

The AKT has a Big Brother (think George Orwell rather than Jade Goody) feel about it. You have to surrender all personal items (including watches, bottles of water and wallets), take the test on a computer and have a CCTV camera trained on you! Try to smile.

Logistics

- You apply online for the October, January or May sitting of the AKT via the RCGP website. As the examination tests how you apply knowledge in primary care, you are strongly advised to take it when you have reasonable primary care experience, ie, during your GPStR year.

- The examinations are performed throughout the UK at test centres run by a company called Pearson VUE, who specialize in computer-based testing (www.pearsonvue.co.uk).

- If you are likely to need extra time because of a disability, you need to declare your reasons when you apply and ask for an afternoon test.

- There is no limit to the number of times that you can attempt the AKT. However, once you have passed you must successfully complete the other modules of the nMRCGP examination within 3 years.

On the day

- Take two forms of identification that contain your signature, one of which must have a photograph (eg, driving licence and credit card).

- Fortunately you are allowed to wear clothes, but you must leave everything else outside the examination room. You can leave for the lavatory or for a drink of water, but extra time is not added. Your valuables can be locked away.

- The examination is taken on a computer (without a USB port to slip in the memory stick that you've hidden in your sock), but you have an erasable whiteboard to scribble notes on.

- When you have finished, a review screen pops up with the questions that you've completed marked as complete, the questions that you haven't answered marked as incomplete and the questions that you want to look at again marked as review.

Preparing for clinical questions

The initial relief of seeing that the AKT is a straightforward MCQ test will soon be tempered by the fact that it can also be the most difficult component to prepare for. The CSA and WPBA are time-consuming and multifaceted, but at least your trainer will be guiding you through a well-rehearsed route and helping you to prepare. With the AKT you are on your own, and you have to plan for an examination that covers 'the whole of medicine'. How best to do it? Simply follow the seven steps below...

1. Don't panic – you're amazing!

Be reassured that sitting down with a huge textbook or a forest-flattening, carbon-bursting printout on 'common problems in general practice' is a complete waste of time. This examination is practical, clinically relevant and based on knowledge that you mostly already possess.

Consider this: you don't suddenly stop in the middle of a clinic and think "Oh no, what if osteoporosis comes up in my next patient, I haven't revised it," and then race to your computer to swot it up it "just in case it comes up". Of course you don't. You manage whatever problem 'comes up' next in your clinic efficiently and effectively based on the knowledge base and problem-solving skills that you already have. If the consultation identifies a knowledge gap, you subsequently fill it. This is the way you work every day. You successfully manage clinics every day in which absolutely any possible problem, real or imagined, that humanity can muster could potentially 'come up' in your next consultation. Just reflect on that for a minute – it really is incredible.

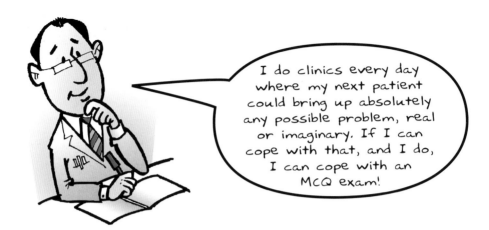

You can cope with any possible problem that humanity can muster. It may be by referral, by subsequently finding further information, by watchful waiting or by reflection and subsequent review but you cope with the consultation and the immediate problem it presents. So, it's official: you're amazing! You already possess an excellent knowledge base and problem-solving skills. If you can cope with humanity's problems in a morning clinic, and you do, then with sensible preparation and practise you will pass the AKT with ease.

2. Identify gaps in your knowledge and experience

As they say, specialists know more and more about less and less until they know everything about nothing, whilst GPs know less and less about more and more until we know nothing about everything. The aim here is to find the point just before we reach 'nothing'! The examination mirrors real-life general practice in that breadth of knowledge is more important than depth. The questions are drawn from across the whole range of medicine. The list of potential subject areas (see page 21) is so extensive that at first sight it can seem unhelpful and intimidating. How can you revise everything from genetics to ophthalmology? As a useful starting point, just looking through and thinking about the list can help you to identify the gaps in your knowledge and experience. If you have recently done a genitourinary medicine attachment then your understanding of sexual health should be fine, but how are you on eyes? Look through the list on page 21 and score your confidence level from 1 (no idea) to 10 (very confident) and then try to focus on improving your weak areas.

3. Use an experiential, self-directed and needs-based learning strategy

Learning works best when it is based on real experiences, is self-directed and is focussed on something that you need (ie, relevant to your work). Remember that the AKT is testing your ability to apply your knowledge in clinical scenarios. Since you are swamped with these every day, there is no need to look anywhere other than your own clinics for revision material. You can devise your learning based around your own consultations, placing emphasis on the

Subject area	My confidence level (1–10)
Administration/health information	
Evidence-based medicine/critical appraisal	
Health promotion	
Genetics in primary care	
Care of acutely ill people	
Care of children and young adults	
Care of older adults	
Women's health	
Men's health	
Sexual health	
Cancer and palliative care	
Mental health	
Learning disabilities	
Cardiovascular problems	
Digestive problems	
Drug and alcohol problems	
ENT and facial problems	
Metabolic problems	
Neurological problems	
Respiratory problems	
Rheumatology, musculoskeletal problems and trauma	
Skin problems	
Eye problems	
Anaemia/blood problems	
Kidney problems	

gaps that you have now identified and using high-quality evidence. To do this, take real-life scenarios and problems and then research the answers. Look for answers using the same evidence sources that the examiners use for the AKT. These are high-quality, preappraised and regularly updated sources of evidence, including:

- *BMJ Clinical Evidence* guidelines from the National Institute for Health and Clinical Excellence (NICE), Scottish Intercollegiate Guidelines Network (SIGN) and other national bodies, eg, the British Thoracic Society and the British Hypertension Society *Cochrane* reviews

Other useful sources of preappraised evidence are the TRIP (*Turning Research Into Practice*) database and the *NHS Clinical Knowledge Summaries*. All of these are, of course, freely available through the NHS library (www.library.nhs.uk). Don't waste time by doing an unfiltered search on PubMed, Medline or Google or diving into the *Oxford Textbook of Medicine* unless you fail to find the information using one of these prefiltered sources. You can greatly improve your search efficiency by 'bookmarking' these resources. If you use different computers at work, personalise an Internet-based bookmark facility such as www.myhq.com or www.ikeepbookmarks.com. Devise a template to use when researching problems – we have suggested one below, but feel free to come up with your own. Once you get into the rhythm this becomes an amazingly quick, evidence-based and effective way to learn. If you just do one or two problems a day then you will have soon revised a lot of information.

Suggested template for needs-based learning

Clinic scenario: 44-year-old man with attack of cluster migraine

Problems: Best treatment? Prophylaxis? Likely triggers?

Answers:

Source:

For advice on preparing for the nonclinical subjects, administration and EBM, see 'Preparing for nonclinical questions' later in this chapter.

4. Keep up to date

The above method works well for learning and answering clinical queries. But you also need to keep up to date with new developments. Be familiar with emerging hot topics in the literature and new research papers that change practice and are considered seminal trials. The gold standard is to do your own weekly review of the main GP journals, but this is very time consuming. There are a number of more efficient methods open to you:

- Subscribe to a preappraised, evidence-based and filtered summary service (eg, *Essential Evidence Plus, BMJ Updates, Evidence Based Medicine*).

- Register for a free 'journal watch' service such as those provided by the RCGP, www.doctors.net.uk and the World Organization of Family Doctors (www.globalfamilydoctor.com).

- Create or attend a weekly journal club.

- Attend a reputable hot-topics or similar course that scans and summarizes the recent evidence, guidelines and developments for you.

The AKT places emphasis on the *BMJ*, *Drug and Therapeutics Bulletin* and the *British Journal of General Practice*, so keep an eye on these for clinically relevant papers and reviews.

5. Be familiar with the major guidelines

If you are to revise anything specific, rather than problem based, then make it the major national guidelines on clinical topics (ie, guidelines issued by NICE, SIGN and national bodies such as the British Hypertension Society). These feature heavily in the AKT. If a major new guideline on a GP-relevant topic (eg, the NICE 2008 guidelines on core treatments for osteoarthritis, or the diagnosis and management of irritable bowel syndrome) has been published recently it is very likely to appear in the AKT. These guidelines are long and complex documents. You need to tease out the essential bits that are most likely to be relevant to primary care management.

6. Practise MCQs!

A famous golfer once putted a 16-foot shot. "Wow, that was lucky," called someone from the crowd. The golfer calmly retrieved his ball and said, "Yeah, it was. But the funny thing is, the more I practise the luckier I get". It is well established that practising questions improves scores. MCQ books are available, but be aware that some of these are based on the old examination, which had a wider range of question formats and was set at a harder level. If you try these and get depressed, do the demonstration examination on the RCGP website and you will feel better! Given that the examination is taken on a computer you should also practise with some online modules.

Subscription-based question banks and 'mock examinations' are available on the Internet and are of variable quality. Highly recommended, and free to British Medical Association members, are the BMJ Learning modules (www.learning.bmj.com). Some of the modules have been specially developed for GPStRs, and are based around clinical scenarios and problems very much as they are in the AKT. They are also quick and fun to do. The modules linked to NICE guidelines are particularly useful. Look for modules covering the areas where you have identified a knowledge or experience gap. The RCGP Scotland has developed an online AKT of 150 questions that cross the curriculum and are in the AKT format. It has the advantage that it is RCGP approved, but it is expensive (available from www.rcgp.org.uk).

7. Make it fun and relax!

Find your preferred learning style (alone or in a group? Paper or computer? Problem or subject based? Telly on or off? Home or pub?) and make it fun. But at the same time, make sure that you don't just concentrate on your pet subjects. If you recoil when looking at genetics, sadly it means that you really do need to look at it. Importantly, you need to relax and give your mind space. GPs have to embrace uncertainty, ambiguity and paradox. We look through a glass darkly and we tinker our way towards the truth, whatever that may be, using intuitive subconscious thought. Fascinating research in cognitive science tells us that to let this part of our mind blossom and grow, we need to make sure that we don't suffocate it; it needs room to breathe. So, keep the right balance. Keep yourself fit, healthy and happy, and don't work too hard. Go for walks, look at paintings, watch films, read novels, laugh. You do not need to cram, stay up all night, take caffeine tablets or miss your sister's wedding to pass this examination.

Preparing for nonclinical questions

Although the vast majority of the AKT is based on clinical medical scenarios, an important minority is based on administration, management and ethics (10%) and CrAp/EBM (10%). Candidates often score lower on these questions, but they are relatively easy to prepare for and you can pick up easy marks here.

Administration, management and ethics

Yes, we know, this subject (with the notable exception of ethics) bores us stupid too. But every job has its 'boring but need to know' bits and general practice fortunately has very few. Even James Bond has to do paperwork and understand the politics of MI6. These issues will come up during your GPStR year and are best covered as they appear, or by identifying a knowledge gap from the list below and requesting a tutorial with the Practice Manager or most appropriate partner. You will be able to add to this list as issues arise throughout your GPR year. *BMJ Learning* has excellent interactive modules, in a very similar format to the AKT, on some of these subjects. Obvious issues to review include:

- NHS structure and function (eg, Primary Care Trusts and commissioning of services)

- NHS political 'hot topics' (eg, Lord Darzi's review of the NHS and the role of polyclinics and private providers of primary care)

- the GP contract, including Enhanced Services, Quality and Outcomes Framework criteria and the 'business' side of general practice

- professional regulation (the General Medical Council [GMC] and revalidation)

- sickness certification and disability allowances

- fitness to drive

- death certification

- the NHS complaints procedure

- access to medical records and the Data Protection Act

- notifiable diseases

- types of prescriptions and the controlled drug regulations

- risk management (reducing the risk of medical errors) and health and safety

- ethical issues

Ethical issues are of great importance and impinge on every working day of a GP. They are rightly given a lot of emphasis by the RCGP. Examples of common ethical problems include consent, confidentiality, applying ethical frameworks, understanding values, assessing mental capacity and the consideration of personal beliefs. The GMC document *Good Medical Practice* is essential reading both for daily practice and the exam. This area is so important that we discuss it in more detail in **Appendix 2: Ethics, Mental Capacity and Values-Based Practice.**

Research, evidence-based medicine and critical appraisal

One of the most refreshing and welcome things about the nMRCGP examination is that the RCGP has cut the CrAp relative to the old examination. This does not diminish the value of EBM in any way – indeed, the importance of GPs engaging in evidence-based practice (as it is increasingly called) is emphasised both in the curriculum and in the GMC's Duties of a Doctor document. Rather, this reflects a change in approaches and attitudes about exactly **how** EBM should be practised in primary care. During the last decade, GPs were taught a lot of CrAp. For a small minority, this was a welcome distraction from talking to patients. For many more, taking time away from patients to search for primary material and then critically assess a linear regression analysis seemed like ivory-tower nonsense divorced from the realities of primary care. The current consensus is that it is important to have some rudimentary statistical skills, but it is not realistic or desirable for GPs to always search for and critically appraise primary evidence from scratch. Wherever possible, we should use preappraised, prefiltered 'secondary' material instead.

Those of you with previous experience of CrAp or who regularly practise EBM will have no problems with this section of the AKT. For many GPs, however, this area represents a knowledge black hole that they have little interest or motivation in exploring. If this sounds like you, please read **Appendix 1: My First Guide to EBP and CrAp**. It is also important to understand the basic principles of audit and how quality of care is assessed (see 'Resources' later in this chapter).

Question formats

The AKT questions generally consist of a theme (eg, low back pain) followed by a question, or a series of questions, related to that theme. For example, there might be three successive questions on low back pain with different scenarios and problems presented. The questions are asked in the following six formats…

1. Single best answer

The vast majority of questions are single best answer. There is a stem, a list and only one right answer, although the other options might sound plausible. For example:

Theme: offspring of celebrities

The name of Posh and Becks' first child is which of the following? (Select the **single** best answer.)

Option list

    A. Bracknell

    B. Burnley

    C. Basingstoke

    D. Brooklyn

    E. Queens

(The answer is D.)

2. Extended matching question

Another common format. A theme is chosen and you then have to match a scenario to a list of options. For example:

Theme: TV presenters

Option list

    A. Chris Tarrant

    B. Ant and Dec

    C. Gary Lineker

    D. Sîan Lloyd

E. Dermot O'Leary

F. Cilla Black

G. Davina McCall

Instruction

For each show described select the single most likely presenter. Each option may be used once, more than once or not at all.

Item

1. "It's day 44, and the housemates are arguing over the shopping list."

2. A panel of judges whittle down a host of aspiring pop stars to 10 acts. Then the public are left to decide...

3. "No! No! No! Not him... He's DISGUSTING! Choose number 3! NUMBER 3!"

   "And now, here's our Graham..."

If more than one option sounds possible then you must select the **single most likely option**. *(The answers are: 1 G, 2 E, 3 F.)*

3. Table/algorithm completion

This type of question tests your knowledge of management guidelines, which are often presented in algorithm form. The algorithm questions can appear very 'busy' on the screen and are conceptually more complex. Take more time on these and read the whole algorithm very carefully before filling in any responses. For example:

Theme: urinary tract infection (UTI) in childhood

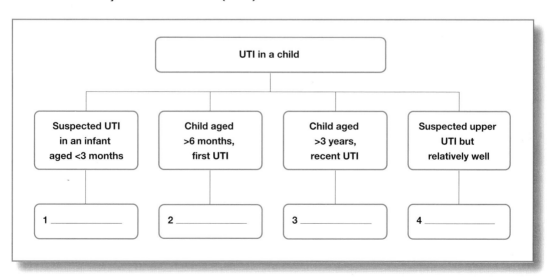

Instruction

For each of the numbered gaps above select one option from the list below to complete the algorithm, based on current evidence. Each option may be used once, more than once or not at all.

Option list

A. Refer immediately to paediatrics

B. Refer for micturating cystourethrogram

C. Arrange urgent renal tract ultrasound

D. Arrange non-urgent ultrasound scan and keep on antibiotic prophylaxis until scan

E. Start 10 day course of antibiotics and observe in community

F. Refer for ultrasound scan within 6 weeks, routine prophylaxis not required

G. Start 3 day course of antibiotics, no further imaging/treatment necessary

H. Start antibiotic prophylaxis immediately

(The answers are: 1 A, 2 G, 3 F, 4 E. Source: NICE 2007 Clinical Guideline, Urinary Tract Infection In Children.)

4. Picture format

This type of question is obviously more likely to feature dermatology (so a quick flick through some 'common rash' pictures may be worthwhile!) than mental health, but you never know... For example:

Theme: unusual neckwear

What is the single most likely reason for the man in the picture to be wearing a neck brace?

Option list

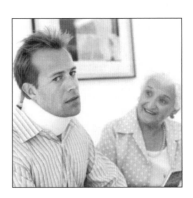

A. As a fashion statement

B. To defend against vampire attacks

C. To support his spinal cord and head after an injury

D. To fake injury in order to avoid attending a blind date set up by his matchmaking mother

E. To prevent injury whilst watching tennis tournaments

F. To hide his tattoo from his mother

(The answer is C.)

5. Data interpretation

This question type obviously mostly applies to the EBM and statistical questions. You may be shown some trial results and asked to interpret them. For example, is a value within a given confidence interval statistically significant? What do the results of a forest plot mean? You may be given a table of data or trial results and asked to make simple calculations such as number needed to treat (NNT) or a sensitivity and specificity. Rest assured that, since you are not allowed calculators, any calculations will be very simple. See **Appendix 1: My First Guide to EBP and CrAp** for guidance on the things you are likely to be asked and how to answer them. Alternatively you may be shown individual patient data (eg, a series of PEFRs, or a spirometry result) and asked to interpret them. These questions could obviously appear as either a single best answer or an extended matching question. For example:

Theme: warfarin versus aspirin in an elderly primary care population

The BAFTA (Birmingham Atrial Fibrillation Treatment of the Aged) study [Mant J et al. *Lancet* 2007;370:493–503.] recruited an elderly, primary care population (973 patients aged >75 years) with atrial fibrillation. They were randomized to aspirin or warfarin. Absolute annual event rates (strokes, haemorrhages and emboli) were 1.8% in the warfarin group and 3.8% in the aspirin group. What is the NNT over 1 year to prevent a stroke with warfarin compared to aspirin? (Select the single best answer from the following list.)

Option list

A. 10

B. 5

C. 2

D. 50

E. 25

(The answer is 50. The absolute risk reduction is 2%, the reciprocal of this is 50. See **Appendix 1: My First Guide to EBM and CrAp** *for simple statistics).*

6. Seminal trials

This is a new question format that specifically tests knowledge on 'seminal trials'. These are key studies that change practice. However, how you define what is a 'seminal' or 'practice-changing' paper remains, of course, very subjective. A valid criticism of EBM is that numbers appear objective, but how they are interpreted remains prone to very individual and human prejudices and preconceptions! A *BMJ* paper from some years ago, perfectly entitled "Seeing what you want to see in randomised controlled trials", pointed out how different doctors can look at the same set of 'objective' data and come to very individual conclusions as to what the data actually mean in clinical practice! However, an awareness of **what are generally accepted** as seminal papers is obviously important here. Recent examples might include the WHI (Women's Health Initiative) study looking at hormone-replacement therapy, the ALLHAT (Antihypertensive and Lipid-Lowering Treatment to Prevent Heart Attack Trial) and ASCOT (Anglo-Scandinavian Outcomes Trial) studies in hypertension, the TORCH (Towards a Revolution in Chronic Obstructive Pulmonary Disorder) study in chronic obstructive pulmonary disorder and the MRC–CUBE trial in dyspepsia. See 'Keep up to date' earlier in this chapter for guidance on how to keep abreast of these. Also keep an eye out for the *BMJ* 'Change Page' series which covers practice-changing papers. Questions could then be asked in a single best answer or extending matching question format. For example:

Seminal trial

The UKPDS (UK Prospective Diabetes Study) for type 2 diabetes showed that (select the single best true answer from the following list):

Option list

A. Tight blood glucose control significantly improves mortality

B. Glitazones increase mortality

C. Oral hypoglycaemics are associated with a significant reduction in small-vessel complications, with an approximate annual NNT of 10 patients

D. Metformin significantly reduces mortality in overweight patients

E. Blood pressure control is not associated with favourable outcomes

(The answer is D.)

Examination tips

OK, so you've prepared. The day has come. You are at the Pearson VUE test centre, stripped to your undies in front of the CCTV and ready to go in and meet your computer. Here are our tips for making the most of your huge potential!

- Think about the answer before looking at the options. If you know the answer before you are 'led' by the suggested responses then your choice is more likely to be right. Look for clues to a diagnosis in the wording of the question; the examiners will not have included irrelevant words.

- Read through all of the responses carefully before answering. It may be that the first response is a correct answer and the urge to sigh with relief and tick it is strong, but maybe the fourth response is the single best correct answer? Don't dive in too soon.

- If asked about the frequency with which an event occurs, look carefully at the terminology that has been used. General guidelines are:

  - *Pathognomonic*, *diagnostic*, *characteristic* and *in the vast majority* suggest that the event occurs at least 90% of the time.

  - *Typically, frequently, significantly, commonly* and *in a substantial majority* suggest that it occurs at least 60% of the time.

  - *In the majority* and *in the minority* mean more or less than 50%, respectively.

  - *Low chance* and *in a substantial minority* mean less than 30%.

  - *Has been shown, recognised* and *reported* mean that there is published evidence of the event.

- Remember, the examination is testing your knowledge of evidence-based best practice, which is not necessarily the same as how things are done down your way. For example, should all elderly Asian or African patients with nonspecific aches and pains have their vitamin D levels tested? The answer is yes, even though your local laboratory told you last week that it was too expensive and a waste of time. The evidence tells us that vitamin D insufficiency is common, symptomatic and reversible in this patient group, and testing has been recommended in several recent publications.

- In some case scenarios it will be very difficult to choose the single best response. Think hard about what should be **accepted best practice**, which might not necessarily be what you have been taught in a tutorial.

- Don't waste too much time on an individual question. Each question is worth the same one point. If you are really stuck then it's likely that the rest of the room is as well. Go with your gut feeling and move on. Research tells us that your first hunch is likely to be the correct answer. Time management is obviously crucial; keep an eye on the clock and your progress through the test at all times.

- If you really have no idea, just guess and go. Remember that there is no negative marking. But, before guessing, first eliminate the answers that you know are false and then step inside the examiner's head. Which answer has the examiner spent more time clarifying? Which one seems to stick out a bit? Which one shares language with the stem? Have a go and move on.

- When the review screen comes up at the end, don't be tempted to go back and change your answers unless you are very sure that you made a mistake. Research tells us that the answer you thought was right the first time is most likely to be correct.

Conclusion

The AKT examination is a good and fair test of the knowledge that underpins the work that we do. If you are interested in the problems that patients bring to GPs then this examination is enjoyable to prepare for and easy to pass. Remember the mantra: **the nMRCGP examination is straightforward, as long as you can see the wood for the trees.** The overwhelming emphasis is on clinical scenarios and how you apply your knowledge in the consulting room, so this is where you should base your preparation. Practising MCQs before the examination is essential and, given that the AKT is taken on a computer, we recommend that you practise using online modules.

Resources

For essential information and sample questions:
www.rcgp.org.uk/the_gp_journey/nmrcgp/akt.aspx and www.rcgp-curriculum.org.uk/nmrgcp/akt/presentations.aspx.

For free online modules in a style similar to that of the AKT:
www.BMJLearning.com and www.doctors.net.uk.

For more on letting your mind blossom and grow:
Claxton G. *Hare Brain Tortoise Mind.* London: Fourth Estate, 1997.

And here's a recap of all of the other resources mentioned in this chapter:

National Library for Health:
www.library.nhs.uk

TRIP Database:
www.tripdatabase.com

BMJ Clinical Evidence:
www.clinicalevidence.bmj.com

Essential Evidence Plus (formerly known as InfoPOEMS):
www.essentialevidenceplus.com

BMJ Updates:
www.bmjupdates.com

Evidence Based Medicine Online:
www.ebm.bmj.com

RCGP Journal Watch:
www.rcgp.org.uk/services/library_services/journal_watch.aspx

Doctors.net Journal Watch:
www.doctors.net.uk

World Organization of Family Doctors Journal Watch:
www.globalfamilydoctor.com

BMJ Drug and Therapeutics Bulletin:
www.dtb.bmj.com

The British Journal of General Practice:
www.rcgp.org.uk/college_publications/bjgp.aspx

Benjamin A. Audit: how to do it in practice. *BMJ* 2008;336:1241–5.

McCormack J, Greenhalgh T. Seeing what you want to see in randomised controlled trials: versions and perversions of UKPDS data. *BMJ* 2000;320:1720–3.

3. Clinical skills assessment

Overview of the CSA: getting to the heart of general practice

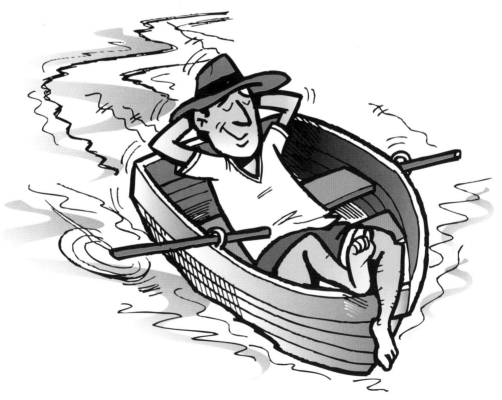

"Never mistake motion for action."
Ernest Hemingway

Introduction

The clinical skills assessment (CSA) is probably the hardest part of the nMRCGP to pass. Perhaps this reflects its importance as, after all, the consultation is the heart of general practice. A full-time GP will have about 10,000 10-minute consultations each year. So you need to hone your consulting skills not just to pass the CSA and your workplace-based assessment, but also to equip you for the rest of your professional life. Good GPs have good consulting skills. Ask any friend or relative what makes a good GP and they, like those asked in various large studies, will tell you it is "someone who listens, cares and understands". This scores more highly than "being very clever and knowledgeable", "wearing a suit" or, surprisingly, "looking like George Clooney/Julia Roberts". Good consulting skills bring job satisfaction. You will find it easier to understand and help your patients, be more efficient and have more fun. GPs with good consultation skills get fewer complaints.

The nMRCGP examination tests your consulting skills:

- directly in the CSA and the consultation observation tool (COT)

- indirectly via case-based discussions, multisource feedback and the patient satisfaction questionnaire

- via the applied knowledge test, which may test your knowledge of some of the well-known consultation models

In this chapter, we'll take a detailed look at the CSA. Are you ready? Are you feeling consultative? Then let's go...

The good news

The nMRCGP examination no longer requires you to spend weeks of your life recording your best consultations, sweating through midnight attempts to edit them with a dodgy VCR machine or obsessively ticking check lists for things like 'cues'. Take it from us: this is a good thing.

The bad news

The consulting module is now a 'live' performance (with actors playing the patients and you playing yourself) and it's expensive.

More good news

The CSA should be more representative of your actual consulting style, and truer to real life, ie, it should test your ability to consult in a way desirable in a good GP. Unlike the old MRCGP assessment by video, it also aims to test your practical clinical skills, which is only right.

More bad news

It takes place in Croydon.

Everything that you ever needed to know about the CSA, but were afraid to ask

What happens? The logistics of the CSA

1. You arrive with the necessary kit and proof of identity, and register.

2. You go to the toilet.

3. You check your fly/bra strap.

4. You are given a 'consulting room', where you will stay for your 'surgery'.

5. You see 13 'patients' for 10 minutes each. Each patient will be accompanied by a trained examiner, who is a GP in real life. Of the 13 cases, 12 cases are 'live' and one is a pilot. (No, not an airline pilot, but a test to see whether it's a valid case to use another time. Your marks for this case will not count, and you won't know which one it is.)

6. Each patient will have their own 'case notes' provided for you to peruse. They will be similar to but less detailed than normal patient records and will be on paper, not on a computer. Any relevant test results will be included. Read these before the patient comes in.

7. The observer/examiner will lurk in a corner with a clipboard, out of your eye-line, marking you. They might interact with you if, for instance, there is something that the patient can't tell you, but generally you should forget they are there.

8. At exactly 10 minutes, a bell will ring, and the patient and examiner will leave abruptly (even rudely).

9. You will get a 2-minute break between the bell ringing at the end of one consultation and the patient arriving for the next. Stretch, snatch a gulp of water and release any pent up energy, joint stiffness or wind.

10. There will be "a short coffee break at a designated time". You may go to the toilet.

11. It will be over before you know it, and then you politely leave.

12. You go to the toilet again.

13. You then have the following options (choose any of the following):

- head straight to the nearest pub to celebrate

- head quietly for home and a good hot bath

- rant to your fellow candidates about what a bastard that actor with 'myalgic encephalomyelitis' was and how it's not your fault that the best part he can get is in the CSA examination

- throw up outside Croydon station

Equipment needed for the CSA

Bring your own doctor's bag. Exactly what you bring is up to you, but we recommend that you just bring what you'd normally use in a surgery or on a visit. A note from your mum explaining that you have lost your kit will not be accepted. If a peak flow meter is left out on the desk, then take the hint and expect to use it at some stage in the consultation.

Types of case to expect

Basically anything, but you are likely to be presented with a mixture of cases that could include (perhaps concurrently):

- breaking bad news

- a patient making a complaint

- diagnosing, explaining or managing chronic disease

- second- or third-party consultation – issues about confidentiality or consent

- a patient with specific health/religious/cultural beliefs

- a teenager

- a child

- a psychiatric/psychological consultation

- an elderly patient

- addictions

- disability – a new diagnosis or ongoing management

- palliative care

- child protection

- concordance issues

- language or other communication difficulties

- a situation involving another health professional

- an awkward patient demand

- a patient with a list

- dealing with a hospital letter, result or report

- an out-of-hours scenario

- a home visit

- a telephone call

- an acute presentation

This list may look a bit daunting, but these are just the sort of cases that you will have to deal with in a normal, if busy, real-life GP surgery. (Although there are lists circulating of cases that have been used in the CSA, we are not allowed to publish these on pain of death and dismemberment by the RCGP). In real life, you don't try to guess what type of patient is going to 'come up' before they walk in, or what particular skill you are going to be tested on – you just get on with it and deal with what comes your way. It's just the same with the CSA, except that someone is watching. What is clear is that you will need to have prepared by doing a lot of consulting, with all sorts of patients, before you take the CSA.

What is being tested?

Here are the domains derived from the RCGP curriculum, translated from 'RCGPese' into English.

RCGPese	English
Primary care management "Recognition and management of common medical conditions in primary care"	Coping with the kind of stuff that presents in GP-land (see **Chapter 1**)
Problem-solving skills "Gathering and using data for clinical judgment, choice of examination, investigations and their interpretation. Demonstration of a structured and flexible approach to decision making"	Find out what's going on, examine and investigate if needed, make a diagnosis and start to manage the problem. Be organised but be flexible
Comprehensive approach "Demonstration of proficiency in the management of comorbidity and risk"	Cope with more than one clinical problem at once, and think about what else might be going on in the background
Person-centred care "Communication with patients and the use of recognised consultation techniques to promote a shared approach to managing problems"	Listen to the patient, find out why they came and work with them to form a treatment plan
Attitudinal aspects "Practising ethically with respect for equality and diversity, with accepted professional codes of conduct"	Be appropriate – in your management, communication, attitude and ethics
Clinical practical skills "Demonstrating proficiency in performing physical examinations and using diagnostic/therapeutic instruments"	Be able to examine and use your kit properly, at the standard required of a good GP
Patient safety	Yup, I got that one…

Golden rules for a successful CSA

Preparation: practise makes perfect

1. See lots of patients.

2. Do joint surgeries with your trainer – note their good (and bad) techniques, and get as much feedback as possible.

3. Ensure that your physical examination technique is up to scratch – are you cack-handed with your otoscope or slapdash with your stethoscope? Can you smoothly examine a knee, a back, the cranial nerves or a chest? Practise with your peers and your trainer. (You may not actually have to examine the patient in the CSA, but you must be prepared to do so.)

4. Look at videos of consultations, using the CSA marking schedule (more on this in a minute).

5. Discuss case scenarios with your trainer and your study group: think about what you might do if the consultation goes in x direction or if you find y… Successful registrars have done a lot of this type of practice.

6. Get used to consulting at 10-minute intervals and practise time management.

7. Work towards feeling confident and slick in managing major and important conditions.

8. Use skill-simulator laboratories if you can.

9. Attend a CSA course, if only to desensitise you.

10. Do role-play – again, if only to get used to feeling like a prat in front of others.

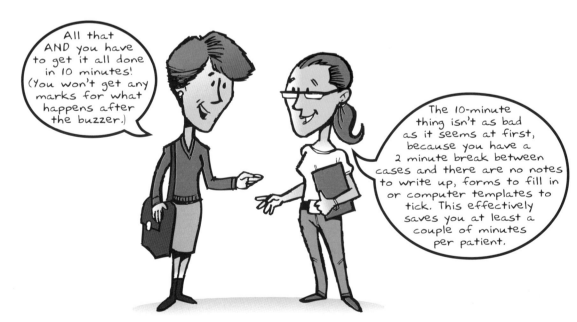

On the day: be cool

1. Turn up in time and in one piece

This is basic life coaching, but we know from past anecdotes that some of you need it. Don't have that extra bottle of red the night before, and do eat breakfast. (Rumbling stomachs and shaky, sweaty hands don't inspire patient confidence.) Leave plenty of time to get to the venue and register (preferably stay somewhere nearby the night before), and relax. Tube strikes and traffic jams shouldn't be allowed to affect your performance.

Remember all of your kit! Charge batteries (yours and your equipment's). Bring identification with you: yes, people have tried to send impersonators! (This is an offence that could get you reported to the General Medical Council.) Wear layered clothing – apparently the air conditioning at No. 1 Croydon veers wildly between tropical and arctic. (But see 'A few don'ts' later in this chapter for what not to wear.) Finally, don't forget your deodorant – remember what adrenaline does to the apocrine glands.

2. Relax

This is also basic life coaching, but remember to make a positive effort to relax both before the examination starts and between each consultation. Take a few deep breaths, clear your mind and be ready to greet the next patient. This, too, is like real life (and is called 'housekeeping' by Roger Neighbour, the guru of GP consulting).

3. Expect the unexpected

It is likely that something a bit left field will appear in this examination. Even this is like real life. There is no such thing as an 'average' surgery.

4. Remember consent, chaperones and confidentiality!

These aspects are being examined too. Remember to bring normal good medical practice into the examination with you.

5. Be curious. Ask questions. THIS IS ABSOLUTELY KEY!

Remember to think broadly about each case. Ask yourself:

- Why has this patient come today?
- What do they really want?
- What is going on in the background?
- Is there something else I should be taking into account?
- Is there more than one thing wrong with them (in real life, almost invariably!)
- Do they understand what I have said to them?

- Do I understand what they think?

- Do we agree?

If you keep these broad principles in mind, the consultation is likely to go well and the patient is likely to help you to help them.

6. Keep your eye on the clock and be ready to wrap up!

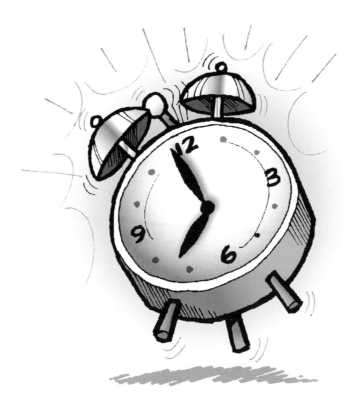

This is a difficult one – you need to be acutely aware of the time, while remaining engaged with the patient. Some suggestions:

- We hear that the conveners have been disallowing stopwatches on the desk, but an unobtrusive watch with a vibrating alarm which you can set to warn you before 10 minutes is up is particularly useful.

- Summarise the treatment plan out loud, including any investigations that you are going to do, and what you are prescribing.

- Check whether the patient understands and agrees with you.

7. Smile!

You are a true professional and the show must go on!

A few DON'Ts

- Don't show any irritation with the patient – remember, they may be primed to be a bit snotty…

- Don't pretend to examine them or turn to the examiner and say "and now I would examine them" – you are being tested on how you really would examine someone! (The examiner may well stop you as soon as you start to examine, and hand you the examination findings on paper – be prepared for this, as it's disconcerting.)

- Avoid lecturing the patient to show how much you know – this is not the point of the CSA and you are likely to a) miss out on valuable information-gathering opportunities, b) run out of time and c) bore the examiner rigid.

- Don't be inflexible (like our bored-rigid examiner). You need to be able to negotiate common ground and put the patient first.

- Don't expose the patient in any potentially embarrassing way during a physical examination. There will be a couch and curtain, as in real life.

- Don't wear anything too flashy or sexy. Apart from you and us (obviously), GPs are a conservative and unfashionable bunch and you don't want to make them jealous or irritated before you start. It might have worked for Sharon Stone, but that was **only a film**.

Practising for the CSA using the marking schedule

Whilst we recommend that you use the marking schedule to assess your progress during training, don't get too hung up on it. Our experience from the old MRCGP video module is that candidates can get paralysed by trying to 'tick the boxes' for the marking criteria as they talk to the patient. The result is a very odd consultation and a bemused patient.

DOCTOR: [*Thinks*] I must check the patient's understanding. [*Says*] So Mr Gargleblast, can you tell me what I've just said, and how you are going to explain it to your wife when you get home?

PATIENT: [*Thinks*] Bloody cheek!! [*Says*] Er, sorry doctor, I didn't realise this was a test…

If you are truly interested in reaching an understanding with the patient, the above scenario can be avoided. This is another example of the importance of our mantra: **the nMRCGP is straightforward, as long as you can see the wood for the trees.**

Marking domain	Competences involved	Remember

Data gathering, examination and CSA
 	
"Gathering and using clinical judgement, choice of examination, investigations and their interpretation. Demonstrating proficiency in performing physical examinations and using diagnostic and therapeutic instruments"
	• Problem-solving skills
	• Technical skills
		• Risk factors
		• Red flags (history and examination)
		• Past history
		• Family history
		• Be curious:
		  – Why has this patient come today?
		  – What do they really want?
		  – What has been tried so far?
		  – What is the effect on their work and personal life?
		• Do you need patient consent or a chaperone for the examination?

Clinical management skills
 	
"Recognition and management of common medical conditions in primary care. Demonstrating a structured and flexible approach to decision-making. Demonstrating the ability to deal with multiple complaints and comorbidity. Demonstrating the ability to promote a positive approach to health"
	• Primary care management
	• Comprehensive approach
		• You have a lot of medical knowledge – it is time to apply it and integrate it
		• If you have a differential diagnosis, discuss it with the patient
		• Make clear what treatment(s) and/or investigations you plan
		• Specify any follow-up plans/time/conditions
		• Manage patient lists actively (see 'Lists and agendas', later)
		• Be curious:
		  – What's going on in the background?
		  – Is there something else going on?
		  – Is there more than one thing wrong?

Interpersonal skills
 	
"Demonstrating the use of recognised communication techniques to understand the patient's illness experience and develop a shared approach to managing problems. Practising ethically with respect for equality and diversity, in line with accepted codes of professional conduct"
	• Person-centred approach
	• Attitudinal aspects
		• Listen and look!
		• Take the patient's ideas, concerns and expectations seriously
		• Be caring and respectful
		• Be curious:
		  – What do they really want?
		  – Do they understand what I said?
		  – Do I understand what they think?
		  – Do we agree?

Like any half-decent cat, you should be curious. The key questions listed earlier (see the 'Be curious' section of 'On the day') are absolutely essential. Practise these basic principles and you should find that you are naturally scoring well on the marking schedule (and, of course, becoming the sort of interested listener that patients want as their GP). Also like any self-respecting cat, even when on a hot tin roof, you need to be balanced. Your consultations should include each of the domains in the table on page 45. The RCGP loves 'domains'. The CSA schedule contains just three, but each one is an amalgamation of some of the competences listed earlier.

Honing your consulting skills

> **PATIENT:** Doctor, doctor, I feel like a pair of curtains!
>
> **DOCTOR:** Pull yourself together!

We all know doctors who are clearly way out in front in the brain-box stakes, but who routinely upset their patients deeply. Your knowledge and clinical skills are important, but how you communicate with the patient matters just as much. Some doctors are naturally good at the communication thing; others have to try harder. We all need to keep improving, which is one reason this job is never boring, but the learning curve is especially steep during the 3 years of GP training. Some great books have been written about the consultation and there are some interesting consultation models (see **Appendix 3**). These models can be useful, but we've seen plenty of GPs-in-training get hung up on their details. They are only tools. Here are a few more key messages about the consultation. These fit with the curriculum and, happily, with real-life experience.

Being patient-centred

What is it?

Patient-centredness in consulting is a surprisingly (and shamefully) new concept. It was first practised as a concept by Balint in the 1960s, originally described by Stewart in 1995, and has now been backed up with loads of respected evidence. See **Appendix 3: Consultation Models** for further information. Bensing clarified patient-centredness as:

1. concern for the whole person, not just the disease

2. facilitating the patient's involvement in controlling the consultation and setting the agenda

3. understanding the patient's expectations and respecting his/her power to make decisions

Why does it matter?

Patient-centredness improves satisfaction, concordance and clinical outcomes. When doctors provide a positive, patient-centred approach, patients are more satisfied, more enabled and can have a lower symptom burden and fewer referrals. (Patients are enabled when they are given the ability to understand the problem, cope with it and make choices about its management.)

Warning: one size doesn't fit all! Whilst most patients prefer to share decision-making with their doctor, some really do not, especially older patients and those with a purely physical problem. Good GPs have the skill and flexibility to judge the degree of involvement that the patient wishes for in different contexts.

> The RCGP curriculum core statement says a lot about patient-centredness. It's a whole (and the first) subsection under *Being a General Practitioner*.
>
> *"A person-centred approach...means always seeing the patient as a unique person in a unique context and taking into account patient preferences and expectations at every step in a patient-centred consultation.... Person-centred care places great emphasis on the continuity of the relationship process."*
>
> *Curriculum for Specialty Training for General Practice. Being a General Practitioner.* Royal College of General Practitioners, 2007.

Concordance

What is it?

Concordance is simply agreement between the doctor and patient about his/her treatment (or nontreatment). At medical school you probably learnt about 'compliance' with treatment. This term, with its connotations of arm-twisting and 'doctor knows best', has been replaced by the more egalitarian term 'concordance'. Because, sadly, traditional hospital training has tended not to allow for the concept of concordance, GPs-in-training often have to relearn how to achieve (and demonstrate) it.

Why does it matter?

The classic example of why concordance matters is that approximately 50% of all medications prescribed for chronic conditions are not taken as prescribed, with significant costs for patients, society and our taxes. Reasons for nonconcordance include religious, cultural and folk beliefs, pressure from relatives, media scares, fear of side effects, cost, lack of information about the condition and its side effects, denial, lack of time with the GP, poor memory, poor eyesight, patient-unfriendly packaging and difficult-to-swallow pills!

How to improve concordance?

This is also simple: be aware of the reasons for nonconcordance and check with the patient what they think about their treatment. You will be amazed at some of the responses!

Starting the consultation – what do you say after you say "Hello"?

In our experience there is no single best opening gambit, but there are some recurrent pitfalls. You may identify with those below.

Opening gambits that may bite you on the bottom

- How can I help? *You tell me, you're the doctor! Har Har!*

- What seems to be the trouble? *Ditto!*

- How are you today? *Well – I've got this cough...* [5 minutes on this, with a dramatic demonstration, followed by] *but that's not why I came, it's just that you asked.*

- I've been checking your results... [followed, after an 8-minute discussion of the results, by] *Well that's fine then doctor, but the reason I wanted to see you was...*

Opening gambits that may work better

- What did you want to talk about today?

- What did you want to see me about today?

- Hello!

- Silence and encouraging smile (but see the warning about the 'smiling assassin' later in this chapter)

- This leads us to...

The golden minute

Beckman and Frankel (see 'Resources' later in this chapter) came up with the deceptively simple technique of allowing the patient to talk, totally uninterrupted, from the outset of the consultation. This often works amazingly well because, of course, most patients have carefully rehearsed what they want to tell their GP. Left to get on with it, they will often come out with a much more complete and relevant history than you could elicit by questioning them over the same duration (usually within 60 seconds). You can then proceed with the rest of the consultation following their agenda, not yours. This reduces misunderstandings and late-arising problems (you know that killer, hand-on-doorhandle moment... "While I'm here doctor, I think I might be pregnant..."), ultimately saving time and greatly improving patient and doctor satisfaction.

(Beckman and Frankel also found that, left to their own devices, doctors usually interrupted patients before they had finished their opening statements and after a mean time of only 18 seconds! Bearing in mind that patients often don't come out with the most important problem first, the chance of barking up the wrong tree once you get going on your own agenda is quite high.)

Body language

Remember to use appropriate body language right from the start to encourage the patient to talk. You know the stuff: open posture, eye contact, head nodding/smiling and mirroring the patient's position. If this doesn't come naturally to you, then look at yourself on video with your trainer and practise specific skills. Caricatures to avoid include the 'nodding dog', the 'smiling assassin' and the 'totally uninterested git who spends the whole time looking at his/her computer screen'.

Questions, questions – an open and shut case

Remember that open questions allow the patient to tell you what you need to know.

"Could you tell me a bit more about…?"

"What is the pain like?"

"Anything else…?"

But sometimes GPs-in-training overdo it – if the patient is clearly presenting with tonsillitis, it really is excruciating and irrelevant to ask them lots of open questions about their pain. Closed questions do have their place. Trust your judgement and cut to the chase:

- in acute presentations
- when time is short
- when the patient cannot express himself/herself, or focus well on open questions
- when you need to rule out red flags

Lists and agendas

Quick Quiz

On average, how many items does a patient have on their agenda for the consultation? (Select one answer only.)

a) None really, they just wanted to check out the new talent

b) 2

c) 5

d) 488,213

Answer: c). On average, a patient has 5 items on their agenda that they would like to address during the consultation.

These agenda items are usually a mixture of symptoms and psychosocial issues, but the social and emotional issues are more likely to remain unvoiced (and doctors tend not to elicit them actively). So, it's official, lists are normal!

Guess how many items the average GP would like each patient to have on their agenda?

Yup, you've guessed it, just one…

This is what highly overtrained educationalists with nothing else to do call 'expectation mismatch'. Some practices put signs up saying "One problem per consultation," which is certainly one way of dealing with the issue. However, it isn't a terribly positive approach and it's a fairly safe bet that it won't go down very well in the CSA.

What the RCGP curriculum says about lists

GPs need:

• to address multiple complaints

• to master an approach that allows easy access for patients with unselected problems. (Translation into English: to be able to cope effortlessly and graciously with patients throwing random symptoms and signs at you in a random order)

• to adopt a patient-centred consultation model that explores the patient's ideas, concerns and expectations

• the skill to manage concurrent health problems experienced by a patient through identification, exploration, negotiation, acceptance and prioritisation

A few tips for negotiating lists

1. Remember, lists are normal.

2. Patients may be more aware of time constraints than we think.

3. If a patient isn't holding a list, ask them if they've got one.

4. Get the list on the desk – ask what they would like you to deal with today.

5. If they haven't brought a list and mention only one or two problems, ask "Anything else?"

6. Keep asking "Anything else?" until they stop coming up with items.

7. Have a quick scan of the problems and decide if there is something serious on the list that should jump to the top of the queue.

8. If not, attempt to agree which problems need dealing with today. Sometimes several items can be ticked off very quickly, leaving more time to concentrate on one or two others.

9. Those items that are less urgent could be brought back next time. Phrases such as "I'll be able to give more attention to this if…" or "I can do more justice to this if…" usually help the patient see that you are trying to help them, not just get them out of the door.

10. If you are feeling overwhelmed by a really long list (our record is 13 items) then say so directly.

11. Habitual long-listers or patients with genuine multiple pathologies should be encouraged to make double appointments, for everyone's sanity.

Hidden agendas

Sometimes patients just won't tell you why they are really there, for many interesting reasons. The patient may be:

*   too embarrassed: "How can I possibly mention that itch in my armpit/jockstrap/other unmentionables? I'd better just start with my (not very) sore throat and see what sort of response I get". (This is a classic)

*   too frightened: "Oh dear, I'm sure I've got cancer. I can't even say the word. Perhaps if I talk about something else the doctor might guess, or it might just go away…"

*   too polite: "I don't think I'd better tell Dr Gubbins that I never took those blood pressure pills – he IS the doctor after all… although I probably will tell him if he asks…"

- too keen on game playing: "Ha! This doctor is really going to have to work hard to find out MY special problem!"

- too limited in expressive ability: "Er... innit... umm... like... dunno..." Teenagers are experts at this approach. Some patients really cannot describe physical symptoms

Breaking the ICE – ideas, concerns and expectations

Most of us learned about ICE at medical school, not just for sprained ankles, but also as part of good consultation technique. The term may be a little overused, but the concept is invaluable during consultations.

Why do ideas, concerns and expectations matter?

- They improve your patient-centredness.

- They help you to avoid falling into the trap of second-guessing why the patient came.

- They help you to fit the answer to the question.

- They help to speed up the consultation.

For example, Mrs Rotten brings little Johnny to see you with his awful cough. You might assume that she wants antibiotics for him. Actually, she just wants to know if she ought to keep him away from her pregnant sister, and knows that antibiotics aren't likely to help him. By asking a question such as "Were you wondering about antibiotics?" rather than just telling her that her son has a virus and therefore doesn't need them, you have the chance to discover her real query and to answer it, leading to a satisfactory consultation.

Looking for C(L)UES

Cues are those little tell-tale signs that a patient isn't telling you everything. Cues may be verbal or nonverbal. They tend to be dropped almost unnoticed into conversation ("...not serious or anything...") and can be as subtle as a sigh, a breath or an eye movement. Cues are clues to help you find out why the patient really came to see you. Like most clues, they are easier to spot in retrospect, especially on video-recorded consultations.

What you do with cues is up to you

Following-up on cues can sometimes open a Pandora's box that you wish you'd left firmly shut, as in the hidden depression that is brought in in the guise of a simple physical illness; you ask the appropriate sensitive question, the poor patient bursts into tears and you spend the next 30 minutes mopping up the tears and distress of many years. However, 3 months down the line, when the patient returns for their follow-up, feeling the best they have in ages, you'll feel really glad you chose to notice that cue. On the other hand, if a patient has a bottomless Pandora's box and loves to pour out their irremediable troubles time after time to anyone who will listen, you may choose to leave some cues unexplored.

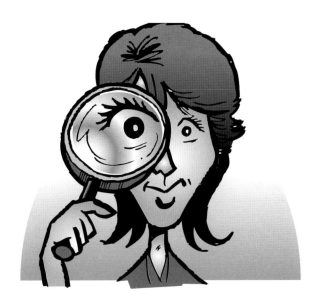

Some doctors become famous for not noticing cues. For them, life is simpler and consultations shorter. Others become perhaps too attuned to cues, digging around compulsively for hidden agendas in a slightly unhealthy way. It's possible to overdo good habits too. There is a law that states that cues are less likely to be picked up on Friday afternoons. There's usually a happy medium. For the purposes of the examination, it will pay to learn to recognise and use cues to find out why the patient really came (see **Appendix 4** for the marking schedule for the COT).

Ending the consultation – it's a wrap

This is a key skill! Somehow you have to find a balance between your caring, patient-centred consultation style and the hard fact that time waits for no one (especially not the CSA candidate). Getting the hang of this early in your career will save you from mountains of angst; take it from those of us who learnt the hard way, floundering in long, drawn-out consultations, running ever later and getting stressed and frustrated, while more senior colleagues finished on time, enjoyed a coffee break and skipped out on visits. We have a few key tips, drawn from hard-won experience and backed up by research.

Say it with words

Wrap up by checking that the patient has understood what has gone on in the consultation and what is planned. You'll be amazed how often this is not the case. Avoid leading questions such as "Is that OK?" and "Does that make sense?" as most patients will instinctively feel the only acceptable answer is "Yes". Some useful phrases are:

- Is there anything you are unclear about?

- Is there anything else you need more information on?

- What do you think about that plan?

Saying goodbye – let your body do the talking

> **What the RCGP curriculum says about ending the consultation**
>
> You should be able to:
>
> • use techniques to limit consultation length when appropriate
>
> • demonstrate effective use of time and resources during the consultation
>
> ***Being a General Practitioner.*** Royal College of General Practitioners, 2007.

Be aware of your body language as you finish the consultation. Just as you used positive body language to encourage the patient's story at the beginning, you now need to use it to signify that it is time to finish – a bit like a landlord collecting the glasses at closing time. This may seem a bit tough, but you have a waiting room full of punters watching the clock, and Murphy's law clearly states that the longer they wait for their appointment, the longer they will expect from you when they get in the room. (There are no exceptions to this rule.) If you have been attentive during the consultation, the patient will not mind you shifting pace. If you have problems closing the consultation, try these tactics, in order of subtlety:

- 'Close' your body language – reduce or cease eye contact, close any notes you have open, cross your legs or push your chair back from the desk. (One GP we know had been experiencing intractable problems finishing her consultations. It wasn't until she saw herself on video continuing to give out strong nonverbal 'keep talking to me' signals that she realised what was happening. She adopted the above approach and instantly solved the problem.)

- Hand over the prescription if there is one (an old-fashioned closing gambit, but still useful). Better still, give them a patient information leaflet – with this you are saying "Over to you!"

- Stand up.

- Move towards the door, pick up the patient's coat/bag and hand it over.

- Open the door.

- Last ditch effort – steer the patient out of the door by the elbow. At this stage you might be feeling uncomfortable, but if you've had to resort to this tactic, the patient probably doesn't read body language that well and is unlikely to be offended.

- All of the above can still be done while smiling, talking and giving off positive signals to the patient.

These tactics work 95% of the time – try them and see. However, there are always exceptions that prove the rule.

Reasons why the 'body talk' approach may not work

- You have not found out why the patient really came. If they had a definite (but perhaps difficult) agenda that you haven't elicited, they may feel that the consultation hasn't even started yet. If they are hanging on, this is a strong, strong signal that something could be up and you'd better find out what. The classic examples are the pregnant teenager, the middle-aged man with erectile dysfunction and the patient who fears they have cancer.

- You have found out why the patient really came but you have not provided the required answer. This can get really tricky. However, asking the questions in the previous sections should reveal what the expectation gap may be and reopen negotiations. Better to have an honest disagreement than a dysfunctional "What was that all about?" consultation.

- The patient is just too distressed to leave. Again, there may be nothing for it but to reach for the tissue box and bite the bullet. Stuff happens.

- Your patient can't read or understand body language. These people may have a sensory disability or a processing problem, as is the case in Asperger syndrome or some personality disorders, where the boundaries and social signals that apply to most of us are not registered in the same way.

- Your patient simply doesn't care about holding anyone else up and is determined to have as much of your time as he or she damn well pleases, and stuff everyone else. In this situation, forget the subtleties and point out clearly and politely that you need to see the next person now.

On a note of caution, Murphy's Law (section 42b, subsection iii) states that if you have just said goodbye to a particularly unpleasant patient and are making rude gestures or cursing behind the door, they will suddenly open said door (to ask "just one more thing") and catch you in the act. Lock the door first.

> Did you know that a patient shaking your hand at the end of the consultation is a sign that they felt that you took them seriously? We wish you happy consulting and many a firm handshake!

Resources

The Royal College of General Practioners website:
www.rcgp.org.uk

Royal College of General Practitioners. *A Guide to the Clinical Skills Assessment.* London: Royal College of General Practitioners, 2007. This DVD and workbook show how the marking schedule works, using 12 example consultations. Use it with your trainer or your vocational training scheme day-release group.

Royal College of General Practitioners. *Curriculum for Specialty Training for General Practice*. London: Royal College of General Practitioners, 2007.

Beckman HB, Frankel RM. The effect of physician behaviour on the collection of data. *Ann Intern Med* 1984;101:692–6.

Bensing J. Bridging the gap. The separate worlds of evidence-based medicine and patient-centred medicine. *Patient Educ Couns* 2000;39:17–25.

Also see **Appendix 3** for details of consultation models and a reference list.

4. Workplace-based assessment

Overview of WPBA: the good, the bad and the ugly

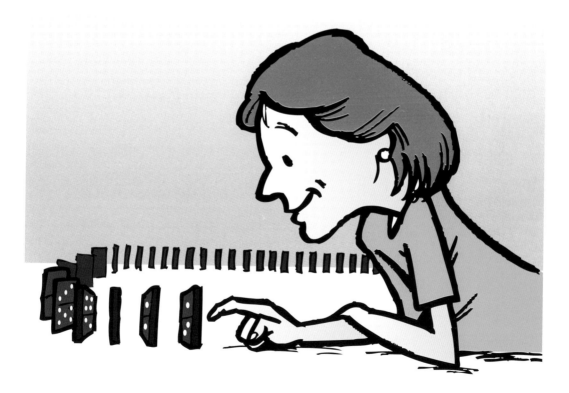

*"There is no limit to how complicated things can get,
on account of one thing always leading to another."*

EB White

The good news

In this module you are examined by continuous assessment over at least 3 years (presuming you enter for the assessment at the beginning of the 3 year Specialist Training Scheme), so a fair and accurate picture of your qualities should be produced (see the 'Magic Eye' boxes, later in this chapter).

The bad news

There's an awful lot of assessment.

More good news

The assessments are 'formative' (about your personal growth and learning) as well as 'summative' (about whether you can perform), so it isn't all about passing or failing.

The slightly ambivalent news

The above can be a bit confusing.

More good news

This doesn't really matter, as long as you want to do well and can see the wood for the trees.

What is being tested?

The WPBA is designed to assess, in particular, those areas that can't easily be examined outside the real-life situation of GP practice. For instance:

- working in teams
- ethics
- professionalism and professional values
- community orientation
- sustaining good communication and good practice
- prioritising and dealing with all types of acute and chronic problems
- awareness of your own health and issues that might affect your fitness to practise

It is a more formal and robust framework for what always used to happen in GP training – that is, a continuous process of learning, teaching and assessment. The difference is that now everyone has to do the same minimum number of similar assessments (this is to satisfy the PMETB that your trainer isn't just signing you off on the nod because he/she likes you).

What happens? The logistics of the WPBA

> **The WPBA asks:**
>
> Are you a reasonable, sensible, broad-based, ethical team worker who can use, apply and integrate what you know, with real patients, in a real practice, alongside a real team, in a community? In other words, would my mum want you as her GP?

- The WPBA starts at the beginning of your 3-year training period for general practice.

- The WBPA consists of lots and lots of little assessments ('multiple sampling' in RCGPese) – see 'Magic Eye 1' later in this chapter.

- Assessments are spread out over those 3 years, in both hospital and general-practice-based attachments.

- You have an educational supervisor keeping an overall eye on you for the whole of your training period, plus a clinical supervisor in each different placement. You will have formal meetings with your educational supervisor every 6 months to see how you're getting on and plan the next stage of your learning.

> **Educational supervisor**
>
> Your educational supervisor (ES) is almost always a GP and has a broad supervisory role during the whole of your GP training. During your ST3 year in general practice, the ES and the GP trainer (see later in this box) are usually the same person; in the 2 years prior to that (ST1 and ST2) your ES may be that same GP trainer, or another GP (this depends on which deanery you are in). Your ES must meet with you to ensure that you are making satisfactory progress from stage to stage, and has the responsibility to inform the deanery if you aren't pulling your weight or are in difficulty. If this is the case you may be referred to the deanery Annual Review of Competence Progression (ARCP) panel (or 'CRAP' panel, as it has been wittily dubbed). Your ES has access to your e-portfolio, and you need them to read and validate your log entries (see 'The e-portfolio' later in this chapter).
>
> **Clinical supervisor**
>
> During each separate clinical attachment you have a clinical supervisor (CS) to oversee your training. This will be your consultant if you are in a hospital department, or your GP trainer during an ST1 or ST2 GP attachment. The CS produces a report at the end of your attachment. He or she does not have the same access to your e-portfolio as your ES.

GP trainer

Your GP trainer (GPT) is the GP you work with during your GP placements both in the ST3 year, and (usually in a different practice) a 6-month ST1 or ST2 post. This is traditionally a mentor–apprentice relationship; your GPT will be closely involved with your progress, especially in that final year. They know a lot about learning and teaching, and want you to do well. They must assess you too, and it is their responsibility to decide (backed up by the formal assessments set out below) whether you are fit to be let loose on the public by the end of your training.

- Assessments are done by yourself, your clinical and educational supervisors, your colleagues and your patients. Some assessments are formal and structured, while others are more qualitative.

- Your learning and assessments are recorded online in your e-portfolio, which accompanies you through all of your placements.

- The WBPA is learner-led: you call the tune, and it is **your responsibility** to get the assessments done.

- Your e-portfolio will be checked at intervals by your deanery to ensure that you are making progress, and prior to its final submission to the RCGP.

- At the end of your training, your educational supervisor will sign you off, using the evidence collected in your e-portfolio to inform their decision that you are 'fit to fly'.

Magic Eye 1: Putting it into perspective

Have you ever looked at one of those 'magic eye' pictures, where the page is made up of thousands of apparently unrelated squiggles? Gradually, as you relax your eyes into a semi-squint and gaze into the distance, an amazing 3D image emerges. The nMRCGP is quite like that – the squiggles are all the little assessments, which aim to build up a 3D picture of you for the assessors over time (don't take the squinting analogy too far here…). Each of the squiggles count towards the whole, but to varying extents depending on where they fall in the overall scheme of the picture. If you try to focus on the squiggles themselves, you lose sight of the picture. In the words of the esteemed RCGP: "The nMRCGP is greater than the sum of its parts".

The e-portfolio

As we write this, the e-portfolio is still very new and is having a few teething troubles. It is constantly being updated and tweaked by the RCGP. Sometimes it crashes. Those of you who are technophobes might need some valium when first navigating it. However, most trainees find it fairly easy to use.

What is it?

The e-portfolio is an electronic log of your day-to-day learning, formal assessments and acquisition of competences and skills along the way to becoming a (new) Magnificent and Really Cool GP. It maps your learning across 1) the curriculum and 2) the 12 nMRCGP competency areas so that you can make sure that, like the trousers on your favourite patient with metabolic syndrome, Mr Carb O'Hydrate, the coverage is broad. The e-portfolio is also the means by which all of your assessments are collated and submitted to the RCGP.

Who owns it?

You do.

Who has access to it?

Mainly you, but your educational supervisor can look at most of it, and the deanery administrators, assessors and the RCGP have limited access to certain sections. Your local deanery ARCP panel will look at the e-portfolios not just of the trainees who are having difficulty, but also of a random proportion of those who are doing fine. It could be you!

Who can add to it?

Again, mainly you, but other people – mainly your clinical supervisors and educational supervisor – can also add to it at various points, generally by submission of assessments (see later in this chapter for more information).

What else does it do?

Your e-portfolio links you to the RCGP website, the GP curriculum, a personal library, a diary and mailbox, and useful resources and educational links. You can book a time for your applied knowledge test (AKT) and clinical skills assessment (CSA), and the results come back into the e-portfolio. It will 'tell' the RCGP Certification Unit when you have made the grade for certification. And if any of this sounds too confusing, you'll be pleased to know that it also has a built-in help section.

What else do I need to know?

Now and forever, the e-portfolio forms the basis of your first general practice personal development plan, your first GP appraisal and your ongoing educational portfolio for the future. This is a Good Thing. (See 'The personal development plan' box.)

Recording in your learning log

Apart from all of the consultation observation tools (COTs), case-based discussions (CBDs), clinical evaluation exercises (CEXs) and so on, exactly what else you put in your e-portfolio is largely up to you (and to a lesser extent, your educational supervisor/trainer. Having said this, it does form part of your material for assessment. In particular it serves to back up your claim to be learning across the curriculum and competency areas, and therefore it needs to contain meaningful entries across these areas (see 'The calculating cat's guide to handling your e-portfolio' later in this chapter). There is lots of room in your e-portfolio to record learning as it comes along, whether this learning is in the form of:

- clinical encounters

- professional conversations (with your trainer, other GPs or hospital doctors and other professionals)

- tutorials

- reading

- courses/certificates (including your day release sessions)

- lectures/seminars

- out of hours sessions

Remember to seize any 'naturally occurring evidence' – when you do something well or come across something interesting, you or your trainer will realise that you've learnt something and you should bung it into your e-portfolio. How much you record is also up to you, but bear in mind that it should be:

- sustainable – see 'The calculating cat's guide to handling your e-portfolio'

- usually broad – across both the curriculum and the competence areas

- sometimes deep – think about what has happened with a patient, in a tutorial or something that you have read that has affected you, and reflect on and write down how this might change the way you practise

- useful and meaningful – don't just add reams of references and lists, but show that you have identified learning points and have a plan to act on them. When you link a log entry to parts of the curriculum, your entry must show how that can be justified

Case study: clinical encounter in ST3 year

You urgently visit Nellie Pickles, 87, after she trips over her chihuahua, Tyson, at home. She hasn't broken anything except the teapot, but you think she might be a bit unsteady and confused. Her medication includes furosemide and digoxin. She refuses hospital assessment because she can't leave the dog. After 55 minutes of negotiation with Mrs Pickles, her neighbour, social services and the district nurses, you manage to arrange interim extra care visits, urgent blood tests and an MSU, a review visit tomorrow and a phone call with her far-flung daughter to discuss her ability to self-care. You arrive back for your afternoon surgery 10 minutes late.

After discussing Mrs Pickles's case with your trainer, you record this as a Clinical Encounter, linking it with the following curriculum headings: the GP Consultation, Patient Safety, Ethics and Values-Based Medicine, Management in Primary Care and Care of Older Adults. Your entry includes your thoughts on what went well, how you might manage a similar case next time and what your learning needs are. On your PDP you enter "find out more about organisation of social services" and "time management".

You realise that you have covered 9 out of the 12 competence areas: 1) communication and consultation skills, 2) practising holistically, 3) data gathering and interpretation, 4) making a diagnosis/decisions, 5) clinical management, 6) managing medical complexity, 7) working in teams, 8) community orientation, and 9) maintaining an ethical approach (respecting her autonomy). You 'share' the entry electronically with your trainer who can link it to these areas (you link to curriculum areas, your trainer validates against competence areas). He or she will add their own comment about what else you could do to expand on your experience or reading from this case, and will finally mark the entry as 'read'. You could then copy one of the learning needs into your personal development plan section.

The personal development plan

You need to put together your personal development plan (PDP), both for your own good (really) and because it will be assessed along with the other parts of your e-portfolio. The PDP is a working plan of your current main learning and development needs. You set targets, methods of achieving them and (satisfyingly) archive them as they are achieved. A few active areas at a time works best, and remember that the acronym 'SMART' (Specific, Measurable, Achievable, Realistic and Timely/to a Time-scale) should apply to each area.

Suitable targets include "Pass the AKT", "Improve my minor surgery skills", "Learn to manage diabetes" and "Set up a study session in your practice on the new NICE guidelines for depression". Not so suitable targets would be "Be pretty good at quite a lot of stuff eventually" (not specific or measurable), "Impress my trainer with my amazing wit" (not realistic as trainers are only impressed by their own wit), or "Plan an amazing stag weekend, in Croydon, just before my CSA" (by definition not achievable, and certainly not very smart).

The calculating cat's guide to handling your e-portfolio

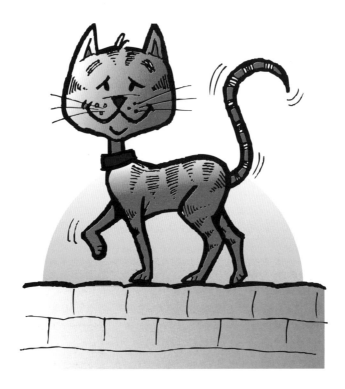

Start early

Cats saunter slowly through life with a clear goal in view (usually tuna). Get logged onto the e-portfolio system as soon as you start your specialist training. Find your way around it and start to record your learning slowly, but steadily. (Warning: those who register late are quickly noticed by their deanery!)

Structure, schedule, discipline

Cats always set aside time to wash their bottoms (usually in front of dinner guests). Set aside a weekly time slot to work on your e-portfolio. This should be easily negotiable in your general practice placements, and most trainees will be able to have protected time in the week for this. In hospital jobs it may be harder to set aside any time, but of course your colleagues in other specialties are studying outside of work hours too. During this time period you should enter learning episodes, check whether any assessments are due, maybe visit a learning module site and so on. Record snippets on paper if you're away from a computer, and transfer them online regularly. Like washing, little but often is much easier in the long run.

Be balanced

As all cats know, balance is everything. Every now and again take a look at the curriculum coverage: have you been going to town on ENT and eyes, but not covered ethics at all? Have you removed loads of moles and forgotten how to take a smear? You need to show broad coverage, which hopefully equates to you being well prepared to handle whatever and whoever walks in the door by the end of your training.

Sharing: not too much, nor too little

(Here we have to leave the calculating cat because cats never share!)

Again, be balanced. Some trainees swamp their (very busy) educational supervisors/GP trainers with stuff to read and approve, while others worry them by staying suspiciously silent and sending them nothing for weeks. Use your common sense and imagination, and choose key, pithy, relevant items to send to your supervisor, thus reassuring them that you are on the case but retaining your ability to see the wood for the trees.

You own your e-portfolio, not the other way around

All cats know who is in charge (them). Remember that the e-portfolio is there for you to show what you know. There are quirks within it that will give you the opposite impression, but you must keep telling it who is boss. For instance, you are asked to record each learning episode in a very structured way, which most free-thinking doctors find as comfortable as a pair of horsehair underpants. We suggest that you don't get hung up on this (ouch). Write what you really want to say, then consider whether the format is challenging you to look at things differently and, if so, add more (or not).

Components of the WPBA

To help get a fair and accurate picture of you, your supervisors are required to use various standardised tools. These are:

- CBDs
- COTs – in primary care only
- multisource feedback (MSF)
- a patient satisfaction questionnaire (PSQ) – in primary care only
- direct observation of procedural skills (DOPS) – in hospital posts
- mini-CEX (yes, we know…) – in hospital posts
- clinical supervisors reports (CSRs) – in hospital posts

These are all fairly straightforward, but we'll look at each in a bit more detail shortly.

The tools times table

Here is the schedule of the minimum assessments required across the 3 years. (It's very exciting.)

Spot the deliberate maths mistake: the reason the last review is at 34 months rather than 36 months is that you have to have everything submitted in time for approval by the end of your training period.

Assessment type	Minimum number of assessments that must be completed by the review at:*					
	6 months	12 months	18 months	24 months	30 months	34 months
Case-based discussion	3	3	3	3	6	6
Consultation observation tool (COT in primary care, mini-CEX in secondary care)	3	3	3	3	6	6
Multisource feedback	1 (5 clinicians)	1 (5 clinicians)	–	–	1 (5 clinicians plus 5 non-clinicians)	1 (5 clinicians plus 5 non-clinicians)
Patient satisfaction questionnaire (primary care only)	1 cycle (only if you do a 6 month primary care post during either ST1 or ST2 year)				–	1
Direct observation of practical skills	8 mandatory, 11 optional (normally done opportunistically during ST1 and ST2 years)				May have to be rechecked in general practice ST3 year	
Clinical supervisor's report	1	1	1	1	–	–

*You cannot carry forward totals from one review period to another, even if you have done more than the minimum number.

My first nMRCGP addition exercise

If you add together all of the above assessments, how many do you get? Choose from one of the following:

   a) five and a half (you've failed)

   b) at least 66, depending on how many DOPS you do (the right answer, and now you can see why we use the Magic Eye analogy)

   c) 6,000,483 (you have OCD and keep repeating your DOPS)

Remember that these tools are objective aids to help your assessors "harvest information" (in RCGPese) and back up their judgement about you. Each one is a very small part of your total assessment for the nMRCGP. Therefore (this is addressed to the perfectionists) you don't need to get hung up about them, but (and this is addressed to the last-minute merchants) you do need to get them done, and do them properly.

Many of these assessments are similar to those used in the foundation programme, so they will feel quite familiar. The main problem you may have is logistical – in your hospital posts in particular you may have to work hard to get hold of people to assess you; be prepared to seize opportunities (see 'Learning in hospital' later in this chapter). The calculating cat's guide to handling your e-portfolio also applies to getting your assessments done – start early, be structured and be consistent. Guidance about each tool is available on the nMRCGP and e-portfolio websites, and you can look at samples of each online rating form on your e-portfolio. In the following pages we give you a bit more perspective and some resources. Now for some detail on each tool...

Case-based discussion

What is it?

The CBD is a more structured version of 'a chat about Mrs Smith', where your trainer has to take on the role of an oral examiner. The point of this is to ensure that you are able to think and reason broadly and justify decisions, under slight pressure, as you will have to do in real general practice. This refers not only to clinical decisions, but also to some of the less well-travelled areas in the curriculum. Ethics, teamwork and community issues are particular examples.

Obviously, the emphasis of the discussion will vary depending on the case and the context (hospital or primary care), but the format is similar. Prepare by reviewing the RCGP guidance. During your training, you must discuss at least 24 cases in this way. The cases should fall across a spectrum that includes children, mental health and cancer/palliative care, and across different settings (surgery, home visit, out of hours and hospital). Good cases to discuss are ones that have taken you outside your comfort zone. Cases that have made you go away and find something out, that you have had to discuss with others, and that have made you reflect on how you practise. You don't have to have managed the situation perfectly, but you do need to be able to show that you are thinking beyond the hospital doctor stage.

Who does it?

You do the CBD, along with your clinical supervisor or your educational supervisor/GP trainer.

What happens?

For each CBD, you must prepare either two cases (in hospital) or four cases (in primary care). Give the notes to your assessor 1 week beforehand; your assessor will choose one of these to discuss. Look through your notes, have a good think about them (using the 'CBD structured question guidance') and bring along copies of the notes to the meeting with your assessor (or have access to a computer). Next, catch your assessor, ie, your clinical supervisor/educational supervisor/GP trainer (see 'Learning in hospital' later in this chapter). If a humane trap baited with chocolate doesn't work, a lasso around the knees can be quite effective.

At the appointed hour, sit down and have that chat about Mrs Smith. It should be like a mini oral examination: you should be prepared to feel challenged and to justify your thinking. The chat should take about 30 minutes, including feedback and completing the rating form, which asks for a rating of I, N, C or E in each of the 12 nMRCGP competency areas (see 'Magic eye 2: get your head around this'). Your assessor needs to complete and submit the form online.

> ## Magic Eye 2: Get your head around this
>
> With the WPBA, most of the components are assessed not by pass/fail standards, but as one of the following options for each competency:
>
> I – Insufficient evidence (eg, in a CBD about managing acute chest pain, your administrative and IT skills may not get a big mention)
>
> N – Needs further development (as the benchmark is "ready for independent practice", then, quite reasonably, you have a bit of work to do yet)
>
> C – Competent (the level expected for independent practice by the end of your training)
>
> E – Excellent
>
> At the beginning of your training, you can expect to score I or N on many assessments. Don't worry, this is OK!
>
> What ought to happen is that you gradually acquire more and more Cs and Es against each competence, so that by the end of your training your educational supervisor/GP trainer can see the fully in-focus, dazzlingly competent you and sign off your WPBA with flying colours.

The RCGP's CBD structured question guidance

Defines the problem:

What are the issues raised in this case?
What conflicts are you trying to resolve?
Why did you find it difficult/challenging?

Integrates information:

What relevant information had you available?
Why was this relevant?
How did the data/information/evidence you had available help you to make your decision?
How did you use the data/information/evidence available to you in this case?
What other information could have been useful?
What were your options?
Which did you choose?
Why did you choose this one?
What are the advantages/disadvantages of your decision?
How do you balance them?

Considers implications:

What are the implications of your decision?
For whom? (eg, patient/relatives/doctor/practice/society)
How might they feel about your choice?
How does this influence your decision?

Justifies desicions:

How do you justify your decision?
What evidence/information do you have to support your choice?
Can you give me an example?
Are you aware of any model or framework that helps you to justify your decision?
How does it help you? Can you apply it to this case?
Some people might argue, how would you convince them of your point of view?
Why did you do this?

Continued on page 70

(All patient data must be made anonymous for the e-portfolio.) You should both be looking to have a broad-ranging conversation which brings out just how brilliant you are at thinking deeply and broadly, so that you can add to your e-portfolio coverage of the curriculum and competences.

The RCGP's CBD structured question guidance *(continued)*

Practises ethically:

What ethical framework did you refer to in this case? How did you apply it?
How did it help you decide what to do?
How did you establish the patient's point of view?
What are their rights? How did this influence your handling of the case?

Works in team:

Which colleagues did you involve in this case? Why?
How did you ensure you had effective communication with them?
Who could you have involved? What might they have been able to offer?
What is your role in this sort of situation?

Upholds duties of doctor:

What are your responsibilities/duties? How do they apply to this case?
How did you make sure you observed then? Why are they important?

Consultation observation tool

What is it?

The COT is a structured way of looking at how you consult, usually using recordings. You will need to have three COT assessments in any 6-month GP placement in ST1 or ST2 as well as 12 COT assessments in your ST3 year in general practice. The COT rating schedule is different from that used for the CSA. The hospital equivalent is the mini-CEX, which again has a different rating schedule. Are you still with us? If you are, well done, because we're slightly disoriented ourselves. If not, go back to 'The tools times table' and repeat the mantra: **the nMRCGP is straightforward, as long as you can see the wood for the trees.**

Over your training period, your COTs (and mini-CEXs) should cover a variety of patients, including children, those aged over 75 years and patients with mental health problems.

Who does it?

You are usually assessed by your trainer, but another trainer (in the practice, or perhaps visiting for your midterm assessment) or a course organiser/programme director might do the honours. It's a really good idea to get a variety of different assessors, as each will have their own views and styles and this will make the process more useful to you.

What happens? (Just when you thought the video had been scrapped...)

Most COTs will use a recorded consultation, but you can also use an observed surgery, particularly if you can prebook interesting patients. If using recordings, choose a consultation that has been relatively complex or challenging, and that you think demonstrates your consulting skills. More criteria can be assessed this way. You must get consent from your patient (guidelines for this are on the RCGP website). You sit down and view the consultation with your trainer, who rates it according to the schedule, again using I, N, C or E for each performance criterion (see 'Magic Eye 2' on page 68), and then fills in the online form on your e-portfolio and submits it.

Desensitising exercise 1: play on your own

Practise filming in your consulting room. Set up the camera in an unobtrusive site, so that it gives a clear view of both you and the patient. Use a colleague to play the patient and get the logistics of filming sorted out (things like finding the elusive remote control, turning on the sound, figuring out that the camera cuts out if left alone for 10 minutes and so on). We've been there and believe us: it's never as simple as filming your sister's wedding.

Desensitising exercise 2: play with friends

Use the COT rating schedule informally with your peers and your trainer before using it 'live'. You will quickly get a feel for what is expected and for the realities of getting feedback, which can be pretty traumatic at first. You will also need this time to adjust to the fact that your bum looks enormous on film and that you have a ridiculous habit of grinding your teeth when you concentrate.

Desensitising exercise 3: "N" = normal

Remember that it is normal to be rated as "needs further development" until some way through your final training year; you are being rated against the standard expected of an independent, fit-to-fly GP. The rating schedule is available on the e-portfolio and nMRCGP websites. The nMRCGP website also has a detailed guide to all of the performance criteria in the COT. We find the guide starting on page 73, written by a fellow trainer, to be even more useful and very practical. A blank copy for you to photocopy and use is included in **Appendix 4.**

Mini-clinical evaluation exercises

Mini-CEX is probably the worst abbreviation in the English language. You couldn't make it up, but someone did.

What is it?

The hospital equivalent of the COT – "a 15-minute snapshot of doctor–patient interaction", according to the RCGP. Again, the problems and settings should vary to ensure that all-important breadth of coverage. You will do three mini-CEXs during each 6-month hospital job. Each mini-CEX will take 20 minutes, including 5 minutes for immediate feedback.

Magic Eye 3: An old model for a new game

The rating schedule for the COT is based on that of the old MRCGP video component. This is complex and looks for quite sophisticated consultation skills. It is not the same as the schedule used to assess the CSA! This is where you need to remember our mantra about wood and trees, and hang onto it for dear life. We make sense of it thus:

- This schedule is a very well-respected model and was too good to throw out with the old examination.

- As the tool is meant to be formative (ie, used for learning, not just assessment), the COT can give you great insights into your current consulting style, and steer you to being much more patient-centred and efficient.

- Remember, too, that as with each part of the WPBA, the COT is not a pass/fail assessment, but a means of gathering information. Don't worry if you score "N" (needs further room for development) on some of the criteria, but do work with your trainer to improve.

- Instead of getting hung up in the horsehair pants of the rating schedule (you'll see this in a minute), think about what we covered in the CSA chapter and ask yourself:

  - Why has this patient come today?
  - What do they really want?
  - What is going on in the background?
  - Is there something else I should be taking into account?
  - Is there more than one thing wrong with the patient?
  - Do they understand what I have said to them?
  - Do I understand what they think?
  - Do we agree?

As in those magic eye pictures, your focus needs to be somewhere in the mid-distance, not on the individual dots (including those that are in parallel with each other, like the COT and CSA assessments).

Who does it?

You can be assessed by staff grades, experienced registrars or consultants.

What happens?

After directly observing you consulting, the observer will rate you using the form in the e-portfolio. The rating schedule is a little different from the other tools, but uses the same principles and more generic headings (history taking, physical examination skills, communication skills, clinical judgement, professionalism, organisation/efficiency and overall clinical care). It was clearly written by yet another committee. You should identify and agree strengths, areas for development and an action plan for each encounter, and whack the form into your portfolio. Simple!

Modified consultation observation tool marking schedule			
Marking schedule	**Evidence (our example: Dr Brilliant, as assessed by her trainer)**		
A. Discover the reason for patient attendance			
1. Encourages the patient's contribution • Attentive listening • Open questions • Nonverbal skills • Exploring and clarifying • Internal summaries • Signposting • Interruptions	Plenty of time for patient to speak, used postural 'mirroring', asked patient to go on and to explain re the "weird twangy feeling in my kidneys".		
	Insufficient evidence	NFdev	Competent · ⟨Excellent⟩
2. Responds to cues • Verbal • Nonverbal • Nonverbal response • Active response • Shows empathy	Noticed and commented on patient sighing "You seem a bit downcast?" Also picked up on patient saying "Of course, my uncle had twangy kidney syndrome."		
	Insufficient evidence	NFdev	Competent · ⟨Excellent⟩
3. Places complaint in psychosocial context • How problem affects patient/family • Patient's occupation	Elicited that the twangs are making patient grumpy at home, and that working in elastic factory becoming more difficult. Also that previously very stressed - "stretched to the limit".		
	Insufficient evidence	NFdev	Competent · ⟨Excellent⟩
4. Explores health understanding • Ideas, concerns, expectations • Curiosity • Discovers health beliefs	"Tell me about what happened with your uncle... Do you think you might have something similar?"		
	Insufficient evidence	NFdev	Competent · ⟨Excellent⟩

Marking schedule	Evidence (our example: Dr Brilliant, as assessed by her trainer)		
B. Defines the clinical problem			
5. Includes or excludes likely relevant significant condition • Gathers information • Attentive listening • Open and closed questions • Appropriate questions • Internal summary/signposting • Pacing of questions • Use of existing knowledge/records • Medically safe	Quite good history and summary of symptoms. Asked re red flags for serious kidney disease. Would checking back for previous similar presentations help?		
	Insufficient evidence	NFdev	(Competent) Excellent
6. Appropriate physical/mental examination • Choice of examination • Mental state examination • Examination explained in appropriate language • Sensitive approach • Targeted examination • Examination addresses patient's concerns	Examined abdo, testes (got consent, explained, checked re chaperone) and urine. Could have asked more about stress/anxiety/depression.		
	Insufficient evidence	NFdev	(Competent) Excellent
7. Makes an appropriate working diagnosis • Integrates information • Recognises patterns of illness • Clinically sound hypothesis • Appropriate use of probability • Can analyse novel/unusual situations • Flexible use of rules and guidelines	Suggested irritable bladder related to stress, especially in view of previous similar episodes. Explained findings normal.		
	Insufficient evidence	NFdev	Competent (Excellent)

Marking schedule	Evidence (our example: Dr Brilliant, as assessed by her trainer)
C. Explains the problem to the patient	
8. Uses appropriate language and give appropriate explanation • Patient-centred • Use of patient's ideas and beliefs • Addresses concerns and expectations • Appropriate timing/pacing/language • 'Chunking' (ie, breaking the information down into manageable bits) and checking understanding • Internal summary/signposting • Varies explanatory techniques • Well organised and logical	Explained normal findings in positive language. "Sometimes if one's nerves are twangy it can feel like the body is too, in your case, your bladder and what feels like your kidneys."

	Insufficient evidence	NFdev	Competent	(Excellent)

Marking schedule	Evidence
D. Addresses the patient's problem	
9. Seeks to confirm patient's understanding • Actively confirms understanding of problem	"What do you think about that explanation for your symptoms? Is there anything else you'd like to ask?"

	Insufficient evidence	NFdev	(Competent)	Excellent

Marking schedule	Evidence
10. Formulates an appropriate management plan • Relates to working diagnosis • Good clinical practice • Appropriate investigations/referrals • Knows limits of competence • Shows knowledge of natural history of illness	Reasonable to order U&E and FBC, and to decide to wait and see. Difficult to score higher here as presentation so vague.

	Insufficient evidence	NFdev	(Competent)	Excellent

Marking schedule	Evidence (our example: Dr Brilliant, as assessed by her trainer)			
D. Addresses the patient's problem				
11. Patient is given an opportunity to be involved in significant management decisions • Shares thoughts/involves patient • Negotiates • Offers choice/options • Encourages autonomy and opinions • Uses time as a therapeutic tool • Balanced plans, doctor/patient-centred as appropriate • Evidence base used	Good suggestions re stress/relaxation, checked if practical/acceptable to patient. Gave patient control about when to come back (pt to choose time within 2-4 weeks).			
	Insufficient evidence	NFdev	Competent	(Excellent)
E. Makes effective use of the consultation				
12. Effective use of resources/holistic care • Understands socioeconomic/cultural background • Recognises doctor limitations • Uses of the primary health care team and other resources • Use of complimentary medicine • Use of time	"What do you think about that explanation for your symptoms? Is there anything else you'd like to ask?"			
	Insufficient evidence	NFdev	(Competent)	Excellent
13. Conditions and interval for follow-up are specified • Safety netting • Appropriate timing • Confirms patient understanding	Good safety netting (double-checked red flags with patient, and told to come back if occur). An open question works better for checking patient understanding than "Is that OK?"			
	Insufficient evidence	NFdev	(Competent)	Excellent

Marking schedule	Evidence (our example: Dr Brilliant, as assessed by her trainer)			
E. Makes effective use of the consultation				
14. Prescribing • Awareness of national and local guidelines • Checks understanding • Checks interactions/side effects • Cost effective • Can justify transgressions • Appropriate use of British National Formulary data	No prescribing this time.			
	Insufficient evidence	NFdev	Competent	Excellent

Table courtesy of David Chidwick, Programme Director, Banbury Vocational Training Scheme.

NFdev: needs further development.

Jargon Busting – mind your PSQs!

The PSQ Guide for Trainees, in the "Help" section of the e-portfolio, makes intriguing mention of "issuing e-tickets" and "capturing" and "releasing" data. Our interpretation:

The **"e-ticket"** is a computer-generated code that is produced, at the trainee's request, from the e-portfolio once the PSQs are all ready to be bunged in to the computer. It is time-limited to 2 weeks, during which the practice has to enter the PSQs online.

"Capturing" – entering the data online

"Releasing" – the educational supervisor allows the results to be seen by you

Multisource feedback

What is it?

This is the lovely RITA by another name. It provides valuable feedback from several different colleagues, which is entered directly into your e-portfolio and fed back to you via your educational supervisor. You undertake MSF four times in your 3-year GP training, twice in the ST1 year (during months 5 or 6, and then 2–4 months later) and twice in the ST3 year (during months 28, 29 or 30, and then 2–4 months later).

Who does it?

Colleagues who work with you and have observed you in action provide the feedback: in secondary care, five clinicians across different job titles; in primary care, five clinicians, mainly GPs, plus five non-clinicians (eg, receptionists, the practice manager).

What happens?

First, fix a date with your educational supervisor/GP trainer to view and discuss the feedback. Next, choose your respondents, then give each one a copy of the instruction letter from the website. Once you have produced these letters, there is a closing date by which the respondents must give their feedback. Let your educational supervisor/trainer know who the respondents are (so that the supervisors can check that the respondents have done it). Your respondents log onto your e-portfolio (they can only input, not read anything) and complete the questionnaire, extolling your many virtues.

Your educational supervisor reads and digests the results, then authorises them to be made available to you on your e-portfolio (the results are anonymous and unedited so, rather than sending them to you 'cold' straight away, your educational supervisor may find a time to discuss them with you with chocolate and tissues instead. You will be able to compare your 'scores' across different attributes to those of your peers, and to view the comments.

You meet with your GP trainer or educational supervisor to discuss the results. Hopefully this bit will be constructive, but you might be surprised by some of the comments and, being the high-achieving, competitive person that you are, you may find yourself feeling wobbly or defensive if not all of the feedback is positive. Remember: 1) if any of the feedback is difficult, your supervisor is probably finding this hard too, 2) if there was nothing for you to improve on then the MSF would be a bit pointless, and 3) if several people have similar comments then the problem is likely to be with you, not them.

The idea is that the MSF gives you points to work on towards becoming an even more brilliant GP than you are already. You can record the discussion with your educational supervisor on your e-portfolio, and make even more exciting links to the curriculum and competences as a result. You can feel the OCD trait kicking in now, can't you?

Patient satisfaction questionnaire

What is it?

The PSQ is a sample of patient views in primary care. It asks about your empathy, listening skills and general feel-good quotient. This questionnaire is derived from research on how patients judge a good doctor, and as you can see below, is amazingly 'touchy-feely'.

You are scored on: "Making you feel at ease", "Letting you tell 'your' story", "Really listening", "Being interested in you as a whole person", "Fully understanding your concerns",

"Showing care and compassion", "Being positive", "Explaining things clearly", "Helping you to take control", "Making a plan of action with you", and a general overall rating. All are scored on a 7-point scale, ranging from "Poor to fair" to "Outstanding". You will use the PSQ twice in your 3 years of training: once in the second half of your ST3 year, and once in any ST1 or ST2 post in general practice.

Who does it?

The PSQ is completed by 40 patients, anonymously.

What happens?

You choose a date. Your obliging receptionists give out the questionnaires and explanatory letters (downloaded from the e-portfolio) to consecutive patients as they arrive, regardless of whether the patients are infants, unable to read English, terminally grumpy or other such irrelevancies (which is fair enough as otherwise they might just try and pick all the 'nice' ones to do the survey). Hand out more than 40 copies of the questionnaire, as some patients will spoil them, not complete them properly, or perhaps eat them if they've been waiting a very long time for their fasting blood test…

Once 40 intelligible replies have been received (we suggest a tick-chart system is used), the survey stops, the questionnaires are collated onto the e-portfolio (by an obliging member of staff, or even you, if you are trusted!) and the results are then looked at by your educational supervisor. The feedback is given in a similar way to that of the MSF, and you can record this as a "professional conversation" on your e-portfolio log.

Direct observation of procedural skills

What is it?

DOPS is a welcome improvement on the old 'see one, do one, teach one' approach to learning practical skills. It uses a more formal approach, with feedback and a rating schedule via the e-portfolio. In these days of specialist nurses, it is scarily possible for doctors-in-training to miss out on honing certain procedural skills such as IM injections, and this system makes sure that everything is covered. We know that some of you may consider this an insult to your years of hard training, but that's how it is, so we just have to bite the bullet.

Who does it?

You can be observed by staff grades, specialist registrars, nursing staff, GPs or consultants.

What happens?

As with the other assessments, you choose which skill needs observing, grab/book an assessor and get on with it. More details are in the box below. Each DOPS will take 10–20 minutes, including 5 minutes of feedback.

Clinical supervisor's report

The CSR is written by the clinical supervisor for each of your hospital posts. It is a brief report covering the knowledge base and practical skills relevant to the post, and also the 12 nMRCGP competency areas. Some of your supervisors may find that this form feels like those proverbial horsehair underpants, and will chafe at the constraints of all those tick boxes. Still, it's got to be done and everyone will get used to it. It is **your** responsibility to get your clinical supervisor to fill out the CSR.

Ideally, the CSR report will be written following a useful discussion between you and your supervisor reviewing your placement. In reality, the likelihood of this happening is inversely proportional to the busyness of your workplace (see 'Give and take – the realities of being a GP-in-training in the workplace' later in this chapter), but you should try hard to have meaningful contact with your clinical supervisor, as many are dedicated teachers and really want to help.

Educational supervisor's review

The educational supervisor's reviews are formally recorded on the e-portfolio and "submitted" with a recommendation about your progress, for consideration by the ARCP panel. The options are "satisfactory progress", "unsatisfactory progress" or "panel opinion requested". Your final "36 month" review comes at least 2 months before the end of your ST3 year. This may also apply to the "12 month" and "24 month" reviews, which will come at least 2 months before the end of your ST1 and ST2 years, respectively, in order for the ARCP panel to consider whether they need to see you or not. (Take the advice in this book and we hope it will be 'not'...) This means that in the second half of each year you have to get your act together and complete your assessments early. You will be expected to have acted on the development points from one review by the time you have the next review (and to have shown this in your PDP).

Clinical skills as categorised by the RCGP

Clinical skills are assessed by DOPS, mainly when you are working in a hospital. The DOPS are recorded in the skills log in the e-portfolio.

Foundation skills

Before you start your GP specialist training you should be completely confident in the following skills:
- venupuncture
- cannulation
- intravenous infusions
- performing and reading electrocardiograms
- injections: SC, ID, IM and IV
- urethral catheterisation
- local anaesthetics
- spirometry and measuring peak expiratory flow rate

You might need to revise and demonstrate these skills again during your GP training.

Mandatory

You should be completely at ease with and well practised in all of the following:
- breast examination
- female genital examination
- male genital examination
- rectal examination
- prostate examination
- cervical cytology
- blood glucose testing
- application of simple dressings

Several of these are key skills, but obviously sensitive. You need a proactive approach as well as patient consent. Get your clinical supervisor to watch you performing these examinations. Attend urology, genitourinary, colposcopy, antenatal and gynaecology clinics when in a hospital, and nurse-led cytology, diabetes and dressing clinics in general practice. Get your teachers to sign you up.

Optional

Most GPs can do all of the following:
- cryotherapy
- curettage/shave excision
- cauterisation
- incision and drainage of abscess
- aspiration of effusion
- excision of skin lesions
- proctoscopy
- joint and periarticular injections
- hormone replacement therapy implants
- suturing skin wounds
- collecting fungal scrapings from the skin (our favourite)

If you are happily cracking on with these during your GP surgeries, then get one of the GPs in your practice to come in and witness one, so that you can 'bag a DOP'. There is no harm in this, the patient will understand that it's a formality, and it's all grist to the mill that is the e-portfolio. Good settings for DOPS include:

- A&E
- outpatient clinics in rheumatology, orthopaedics and gynaecology
- minor surgery clinics in general practice and dermatology and plastic surgery
- outpatient clinics
- family planning clinics

Give and take – the realities of being a GP-in-training in the workplace

Learning in hospital

Every doctor in a hospital training post finds a tension between the service element and learning opportunities. You are being paid to look after patients, but you also have to grasp the opportunity to learn as much as possible. In busy jobs you can learn the key GP skills of triage, handling multiple demands and managing time, while a 'quiet' job gives you more time for reflection and reading. Both are valuable. A few suggestions from your peers and predecessors:

- Learn to negotiate and to be flexible – you are in the job to serve your patients and your employers, as well as to train. A little give and take will stand you in good stead when you need that COT done in a hurry.

- Practise exploring patient-centred consulting and patient understanding, despite working in a more doctor (or manager)-driven system.

- You may find yourself working with trainees in other specialties whose needs seem to be put above yours by the consultants. Again, this is a chance to hone your negotiating skills! Swap into outpatient clinics as much as possible – you may well find that your surgical trainee colleagues would love to spend more time in theatre while you do a clinic for them.

- Use study leave to visit clinics in different specialties to fill in clinical gaps.

- Be organised – keep notes of encounters and cases to enter into your e-portfolio or use for CBDs. Try to make the time to use any formal learning opportunities that are provided by your deanery. Ask to be paged by the postgraduate centre when your learning set (a study group arranged by your local programme directors) is meeting – this works wonders!

- Be politely assertive: consultants may be hard to pin down for performing assessments. They are busy, and some of them trained in an era when learning happened by doing, not sitting down with forms. Find out who your clinical supervisor is in week 1 of any post. Get DOPSs signed off by registrars and senior nurses. When it comes to formal assessments, set up everything you can beforehand – print off the forms, find the case(s), book a room and a time, and then catch your consultant and drag him/her off to do the necessary.

Learning in general practice

We've talked about this in **Chapter 1**. On the whole, educational supervisors/GP trainers are used to assessing their learners in the workplace, and they relish the teaching opportunities. Like most doctors, though, they don't like being told what to do, so they too may chafe at the constraints of all the different forms, boxes, templates, criteria and competencies (or competences or competency areas... the RCGP tells us that these are different, but they seem to be used interchangeably by the RCGP itself). This is why our mantra is so important. These assessments and the e-portfolio are tools to help you and your trainer reach your goal of knowing, doing, applying, integrating and showing your knowledge, skills and attributes. In other words, of becoming a brilliant GP and showing that you are. Each one is only a small piece of the magic eye picture – so don't sweat the small stuff, but aim for the big view. Remember: **the nMRCGP is straightforward, as long as you can see the wood for the trees.**

What if things go wrong?

Although we hope that most of you will find the WPBA straightforward, we know that in real life glitches happen. It is possible that you may fall out with one or more of your clinical supervisors, find your educational supervisor uncooperative or hard to get hold of, feel that a particular assessment is unfair (remember, most individual assessments are tiny pieces of the picture) or find that you and your educational supervisor/GP trainer just don't get on.

First, talk it through with your peers. Other people may have negotiated similar problems and can suggest winning tactics or a different perspective. Try to negotiate. If you are still having trouble, talk to your educational supervisor (if they are not the problem!) or your programme director/course organiser. If a particular consultant is habitually difficult, the programme director can feed this back to them or their department. If you are struggling because of your own health or life events, do tell your educational supervisor or programme director early on – they will want to help you.

Resources

The nMRCGP website and the e-portfolio websites both contain many links to resources for all the elements of WPBA. These are constantly being updated, so we're not going to list them here. Our advice is "seek and (mostly) ye shall find". Your peers are also invaluable resources, especially the geeky ones; we recommend that you cultivate them.

And finally

> **"In my end is my beginning."**
> *Mary, Queen of Scots*

This means two things in this context:

1) **Learning never stops**, it goes round in circles and in spirals and in clever whirly patterns. 'Doing' your nMRCGP is only the beginning, and should set you on the road to lifelong learning as a habit, not a 'have-to'. Our hope for you is that you can enjoy the first steps in this journey a bit, and that we might have helped you in that enjoyment.

2) **Well done, you have reached the end of this book**. Now go back and look at the beginning again, and repeat after us:

The nMRCGP is straightforward, as long as you can see the wood for the trees.

Appendix 1:

My first guide to evidence-based medicine and critical appraisal

Those 'in the know' can skip this bit, but in our experience there are a significant number of GPs who remain intimidated by research and statistics and would like to cut the CrAp (critical appraisal) all together. This section is for them. We are not attempting to teach evidence-based medicine (EBM), just to give you some basic tools for the applied knowledge test (AKT) and hopefully some enthusiasm to develop further. We heartily recommend *Evidence-based Medicine Toolkit* as a light, clear and concise guide. For those who want more flesh on the bones, *How to Read a Paper* is a key text (see 'Resources' at the end of this appendix).

Here are seven steps that will help you to cope with EBM in the AKT...

1. Understand what EBM actually is

Is EBM cook-book medicine that creates a new paternalism of 'evidence knows best'? No. EBM is "the integration of the best available evidence with our clinical expertise and our patients' unique values and circumstances" (Straus et al. *Evid Based Med* 2007;12:2–3) and the RCGP *Curriculum for General Practice* states, "EBM should contribute to patient care but not override it." So remember that, whilst research findings are important, if your clinical judgement or your patient's beliefs are against the treatment then that trumps whatever the evidence says. The classic five-step model of EBM is:

1. Ask an answerable question.

2. Search for the evidence.

3. Critically appraise the evidence.

4. Make the decision, integrating this evidence with your judgement and the patient's values.

5. Evaluate your performance.

PICO is the acronym classically used to ask questions, eg:

Patient or problem: **85-year-old lady with AF**

Intervention: **warfarin**

Comparison intervention: aspirin

Outcomes: morbidity and mortality

The emphasis now is on GPs primarily being 'evidence users' using prefiltered, secondary sources (as discussed in **Chapter 2**). However, if you do not find your answer in those sources then a *Medline* search is necessary. The *askMEDLINE* search service uses the PICO format.

2. Understanding different study types

Different studies are needed to answer different research questions.

Case–control study

Case–control studies are retrospective studies that answers questions related to aetiology. Patients who have developed a disorder, and their exposure to a possible cause, are compared to a control group without the disorder. They are quick, cheap and enable rare conditions to be studied, but eliminating confounding factors is hard and they cannot prove causality.

Example: is mobile phone use associated with brain tumours? A group of patients who have developed tumours would have their retrospective mobile phone usage compared to a control group without tumours.

Cohort study

Cohort studies are prospective and answer questions related to aetiology and prognosis. Patients with a disease, or exposure to a risk, are followed-up over time and compared to a control group. They are relatively cheap and simple compared to RCTs and are more rigorous than case–control studies, but it remains difficult to exclude confounding factors.

Example: Richard Doll's famous study that established a higher incidence of cancer in a cohort of smokers compared to a cohort of nonsmokers. These studies are also useful for prognosis, eg, what is the prognosis for a cohort of patients with early prostate cancer compared to a control cohort?

Randomised controlled trial

Randomised controlled trials (RCTs) are the 'gold standard' for questions related to interventions and are the most powerful way of eliminating confounding factors and bias. But they are expensive, laborious and can still be subject to selection and observer bias. Large numbers are needed to assess rare events and in negative trials it can be impossible to know if it is a 'true' negative, or if the trial was simply too small to show an effect. This can be partially overcome when results are combined in a systematic review.

Qualitative studies

Qualitative studies involve structured interviews and the observation of participants. They can give useful information on patient perspectives and quality of life issues and can help fill gaps in knowledge that numbers cannot answer (eg, why do so many men want a prostate-specific antigen test when there is no evidence of benefit? Why do parents worry so much about coughs?). Although they are qualitative rather than quantitative, they are still designed in a rigorous and systematic way with a variety of methodologies, but bias (particularly related to the agenda of the researcher) is inevitable.

Diagnostic studies and economic evaluations

Diagnostic studies answer questions related to diagnosis by assessing the accuracy of a test, clinical symptom or sign compared to a gold standard control, while economic evaluations obviously assess cost-effectiveness.

3. Having a basic template for appraisal of a paper

A very simple template for appraisal involves asking if the study is both valid and relevant.

Is the study valid?

- Is the methodology sound and are the results statistically significant and clinically important?

Is it relevant?

- Are the results from this study applicable to my patient?

For relevance in primary care there are two fundamental issues. Firstly, is the study looking at an outcome that is clinically important? Is the study patient-orientated evidence that matters (POEM) (a study that looks at clinical outcomes, eg, this drug reduces fractures) or disease-orientated evidence (DOE) (a study that looks at surrogate markers, eg, this drug increases bone mineral density)? Secondly, how applicable is the study population to my particular patient? RCTs are generally done in secondary care. Older, frailer patients and those with comorbidities are often excluded. Two important but ill-understood concepts in appraising RCT methodology are allocation concealment and intention-to-treat analysis. Both are necessary to minimise bias.

Allocation concealment

Have the researchers concealed the allocation of patients from the clinicians? Clinicians are human and if they can tell (eg, by holding the envelope up to the light!) which treatment arm a patient is going to go into, they will distort the randomisation process (eg, by putting safe patients into the warfarin group and risky ones into the placebo group). Allocation concealment is considered the most important thing to look for when appraising RCTs.

Intention-to-treat analysis

All of the patients should be analysed in all of the groups into which they were originally assigned, even if they subsequently switch treatments or never even took the treatment. This is very counterintuitive. If a patient never took drug A, and even switched to drug B, what is the logic of still including them in the drug A group when it comes to analysing results? The answer is that we can only be confident that the two original randomised groups remain comparable if there is intention-to-treat analysis. Without it, researchers could pick and choose who ends up in the final analysis. The alternative is per-protocol analysis, which is known to increase bias.

4. Calculating treatment effects

A basic skill for real life and the AKT is calculating treatment effects in terms of:

- RR: relative risk or risk ratio
- RRR: relative risk reduction
- AR: absolute risk
- ARR: absolute risk reduction
- NNT: numbers needed to treat = 1/ARR
- OR: odds ratio

To calculate these figures we need to know the experimental event rate (EER) (the rate at which an event occurs in the experimental or treatment group) and the control event rate (CER). Typically, the EER and CER are represented in a table like like the one on the next page.

	Control	Experimental	Total
Event	a	b	a + b
No event	c	d	c + d
Total	a + c	b + d	

CER = a/(a + c) and EER = b/(b + d)

RR = EER/CER

ARR = CER – EER

RRR (a percentage estimate of ARR in the control group) = (CER – EER)/CER

NNT = 1/ARR

However, these letters and acronyms make it seem more complicated than it is.

Example: suppose that the CER of a myocardial infarction is 25% and the EER is 20% for a drug over 5 years.

- RR = EER/CER = 20/25 = 0.8 or 80%

- ARR = CER – EER = 25 – 20 = 5%

- NNT = 1/ARR = 1/0.05 = 20

Rest assured that any calculation in the AKT will be very simple. For example, try this in your head. A drug trial reduces the risk of a major event in the next 5 years from 6% to 4%.

- What is the RRR? What is the ARR? What is the NNT?

(Answers: RRR = 1/3, ARR = 2% and NNT = 1/0.02 = 50 patients.)

RRs are constant across a range of ARs, which is why calculating the AR and NNT is so important. If an experimental drug reduces your risk of a myocardial infarction from 2% to 1% then the RRR is 50% (the drug halves your risk), but the ARR is only 1% and the NNT is 1/0.01 = 100. But if a drug reduces your risk from 40% to 20% then the RRR is still 50%, but the ARR of 20% and the NNT of 1/0.2 = 5 are clinically much more significant. As ARs are more relevant to our patients, NNT is considered the most useful measure of benefit. As RRs look more impressive they are used extensively in pharmaceutical marketing. When discussing NNT with patients, the time period is crucial, eg, an NNT of 20 over 1 year is very different to an NNT of 20 over 10 years.

OR is another way of expressing a treatment effect, and approximates to RR. For anorak reasons it is favoured in systematic reviews and in case–control studies. An OR is simply the odds of an event happening versus it not happening. Looking at the above table, the odds of an event in the control group is a/(a + c). The odds of an event in the experimental group is b/(b + d). The OR will then be the ratio of the two. Again, this sounds more complicated than it actually is.

Example: In a trial of a new drug, 500/1,000 patients died in the control arm and 250/1,000 died in the treatment arm.

Questions:

A. What are the odds of death in the treatment arm?

B. What are the odds of death in the control arm?

C. What is the OR of the study?

(Answers: A = 0.25, B = 0.5, C = 0.25/0.5 = 0.5.)

It is possible to convert the OR from a meta-analysis into an absolute NNT, but this is real A-level stuff. You will not to be asked to do this in the AKT, but it is useful for interpreting systematic reviews. You can find guidance on how to do it at the Centre for Evidence-Based Medicine website (www.cebm.net).

5. Assessing statistical significance

This is done using *P*-values and CIs. Most people can get their heads around *P*-values but struggle with CIs, which are actually far more useful.

P-value

This is the probability of an event occurring by chance. For entirely arbitrary reasons, standard scientific practice is that a *P*-value of <0.05 (a less than 1 in 20 probability that the event happened by chance) is significant. A significant result in a trial will therefore always have a 1 in 20 chance of appearing, which is very sobering when you consider how many are published! This is also why you have to be very careful of subgroup analyses in large RCTs that have a negative main result. If an author analyses enough subgroups then he or she will eventually find one with a statistically significant result. Seeing a significant result like this that is not actually real is called a type 1 error. Bear in mind that a nonsignificant *P*-value tells you that either there is really no difference between the groups or the trial wasn't large enough. It cannot tell you which.

Confidence intervals

CIs are cool. You will never have to calculate a CI, but knowing how to interpret them is perhaps the single most useful way to improve your CrAp skills and appreciation of scientific literature. A 95% CI is a range of numbers around a result within which you can be 95% confident that the true result lies. To quote Bandolier, "You can be 95% certain that the truth is somewhere inside a 95% CI." Like *P*-values, CIs are a measure of whether a result has reached statistical significance (and, as for a *P*-value, the 5% cut off is arbitrary), but they also give useful additional information about the precision of a study. When interpreting a CI you ask yourself: "Is the result statistically significant?" and "How wide is the CI"?

A great thing about CIs is that you can easily tell if statistical significance has been reached. **If the CI includes the value that reflects no-effect, the result is statistically nonsignificant.** The value of no-effect will be:

- 1 for results that are expressed as ratios (RRs, ORs)

- 0 for measurements (eg, mean differences, percentages or ARRs)

To illustrate this, look at the hypothetical examples below:

- A study of aspirin versus control to reduce the occurrence of cardiovascular events results in an RR of 0.80 (95% CI 0.70–0.90).

This means that the patients treated with aspirin experienced fewer cardiovascular events than the control group, with an RR of 0.8. The 95% CI for this RR is from 0.70 to 0.90. From this we can infer two things. Firstly, the result is statistically significant because the CI does not cross 1 (the value of no-effect for a ratio). Secondly, the data are consistent with an RR anywhere between 0.7 and 0.9.

- A study of warfarin versus control to reduce the occurrence of cardiovascular events finds an ARR of 3% (95% CI –1.6 to 6.0).

This means that the group of patients treated with warfarin has a 3% ARR in events, but it does not reach statistical significance because the CI crosses zero (the value of no-effect for a measurement).

As well as assessing statistical significance, CIs indicate how precise the result is. The narrower the CI, the more precise the result; the larger the study, the greater its power and the narrower the CI tends to be. If a CI is very wide, the results are less precise and this implies that the study was underpowered or small.

Example: a study reports an ARR of 12% (95% CI 9–14). The data are consistent with a real ARR of between 9% and 14%, so the reported ARR of 12% looks precise. If, however, the study had reported an ARR of 12% (95% CI 2–38) then we could say that the result was statistically significant, but that the data were consistent with a true ARR of anywhere between 2% and 38%, ie, the result is much less precise.

If a trial is nonsignificant, which will happen frequently if the study is too small (ie, underpowered with a wide CI), a common error is to conclude that there is no treatment effect when in fact there is. This is a type 2 error. If a significant effect has not been found, a useful question to avoid a type 2 error is 'has there been a meta-analysis?'

6. Interpreting systematic reviews and meta-analyses: don't lose the plot

Pooling results from different studies in order to increase the power of the study and reduce the CI is valuable for avoiding type 2 errors. A meta-analysis is the statistical technique used to integrate the results of pooled studies. A systematic review involves a determined effort to include all of the relevant studies on the subject, to critically appraise them before inclusion and then draw conclusions based on the synthesis of the data. ORs are more appropriate for meta-analyses, which is why they are frequently used when reporting systematic reviews. The most famous collaboration of systematic reviews is, of course, Cochrane.

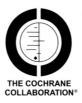

THE COCHRANE COLLABORATION®

Look at the logo. In the centre is a forest plot or 'blobogram', which can be used to represent the results of a systematic review. The logo comes from a famous meta-analysis of seven RCTs in which steroids were given to pregnant women who were expected to give birth prematurely. Most of the studies were negative. But the pooled results narrowed the confidence intervals (ie, improved the precision) and showed a statistically significant and clinically important result: the babies of mothers who were given steroids were less likely to die. You won't have to do anything complicated in the AKT, but knowing how to interpret a forest plot is a useful skill.

Look at our hypothetical forest plot of studies A, B and C and their ORs.

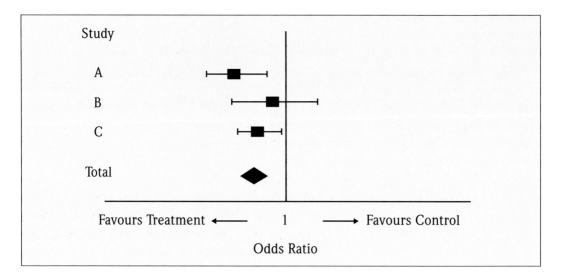

The horizontal lines represent the 95% CIs. The square in the middle of each line is the reported result of the study. The vertical line is the 'line of no-effect', which for a ratio is 1. Anything to the left favours the treatment, while anything to the right favours the control. Therefore, studies A and C are statistically significant because the CI does not cross the no-effect value. The overall result pooled by meta-analysis is represented by the diamond, the length of which represents the CI. As the diamond does not cross the line of no-effect, this is a positive result.

7. Calculating sensitivity, specificity and likelihood ratios in diagnostic studies

To most GPs this is a hazy concept, vaguely snatched at just before an examination only to disappear into the ether immediately afterwards. However, as we become encouraged to do more patient testing it becomes an increasingly important concept to understand. Imagine a new test for chlamydia. The results are presented as:

	Present	Absent
Positive	a	b
Negative	c	d

The **sensitivity** of the test is $a/(a + c)$

The **specificity** of the test is $d/(b + d)$

The **positive predictive value** (**PPV**) is $a/(a + b)$

The **negative predictive value** (**NPV**) is $d/(c + d)$

You are very unlikely to have to calculate likelihood ratios, but the formulae are:

- The likelihood ratio of a positive result = sensitivity/(1 – specificity)

- The likelihood ratio of a negative result = (1 – sensitivity)/specificity

And now in simple English...

Sensitivity and specificity

- The sensitivity of the test is the proportion of people with the disease who have a positive test result. If this chlamydia test proves to be highly sensitive then it will be good at determining who has the infection and there will be few false-negative results.

- The specificity of the test is the proportion of people without the disease who have a negative test result. If this chlamydia test is highly specific then it will be good at excluding people without the infection and there will be few false-positive results.

To help remember this, the mnemonics **SnNout** and **SpPin** are often used:

- **SnNout**: if a test is highly sensitive (**Sn**) then a negative result (**N**) rules the diagnosis **out**.

- **SpPin**: if a test is highly specific (**Sp**) then a positive result (**P**) rules the diagnosis **in**.

Predictive values

Predictive values are very seductive as they are easy to grasp. The PPV is the percentage of patients who test positive for chlamydia who really do have it, and the NPV is the percentage who test negative for chlamydia but do not really have it. Crucially, these are dependent on the background prevalence of the disorder in the population. If a disease is rare, the PPV will be low (sensitivity and specificity remain constant). So we would expect the PPV of a chlamydia test to be higher in a population taken from a genitourinary medicine clinic than from a random sample in primary care. The measure of test accuracy that is most useful is the **likelihood ratio**, which gives an overall measure of the efficacy of the test. Again, for the purpose of the AKT, you will only be asked to do simple calculations. For example try:

	Present	Absent
Positive	30	50
Negative	90	200

What is the sensitivity of the test?
- Sensitivity = 30/(30 + 90) = 30/120 = 25%

What is the specificity of the test?

- Specificity = 200/(50 + 200) = 200/250 = 80%

Interpretation: the test has reasonable specificity, so a positive result can be useful for ruling a diagnosis of strep throat in. However, the sensitivity is very poor so many people with strep throat will be missed. A crucial point in interpreting these diagnostic studies is to know the gold standard that the new test was compared against. Looking at the above table, how do we know that the 120 patients listed as suffering from strep throat really did have it? Without this information, such a study is impossible to interpret.

Conclusion

Knowing and understanding different study types and some simple appraisal and statistical skills are all you need for the AKT. A basic understanding of these will improve your confidence and appreciation of the literature – honest!

Resources

Badenoch D, Heneghan C. *Evidence-Based Medicine Toolkit*. Oxford: Blackwell BMJ Books, 2006.

Greenhalgh T. *How to Read a Paper: the Basics of Evidence Based Medicine*. Oxford: Blackwell BMJ Books, 2006.

The Centre for Evidence-Based Medicine. *EBM Tools*. Available from: www.cebm.net.

Appendix 2:

Ethics, mental capacity and values-based practice

One of the many fascinating aspects of general practice is the wide range of ethical dilemmas we are presented with. The closer you look, the more there are and the more complex they become. So understanding their basic principles is essential for general practice, and thus for all parts of the nMRCGP. Ethical dilemmas are easy to think about when confronted with requests for a termination of pregnancy or assisted dying – in fact, anything related to the innate human preoccupation with sex and death. But many seemingly dull, daily requests have ethical dimensions. Here is one example.

PATIENT: You know doc, that blue 'reliever' you prescribed me just ain't the same as Ventolin. Can you give me the proper Ventolin stuff?

DOCTOR: Uhmm… well, let's see…

The four classic principles of bioethics give a useful framework for thinking these problems through.

The four classic principles of bioethics

The four classic principles of bioethics are:

- autonomy – a patient's right to self determination

- beneficence – to do good

- nonmaleficence – to do no harm

- justice – truth, the law and fairness for all

Let's use these principles to look at our Ventolin-requesting patient. These principles do not, of course, give you a **right** answer, but provide a useful template for thought and reason. You could say to yourself, "My patient has the right to make this request for branded Ventolin and his autonomy should be respected. There is no objective evidence that it will do any good, but, subjectively, if he feels better about it then this may do him good in itself. It certainly will not do him any harm, but it is a more expensive option and will take resources away from other patients".

In the NHS the fourth principle, justice, is often a key factor. The NHS is essentially a utilitarian organisation (ie, it aims for the greatest good for the greatest number of people within fixed resources), and yet the GMC document *Duties of a Doctor* states that we must make the care of the patient our first concern. GPs are involved in a constant ethical conflict as we strive to balance the needs of our individual patients whilst being just to the wider group.

A limitation of the four principles is that they do not explicitly include the vital issues of **confidentiality** and **consent**. Of course, these need to be carefully considered across a wide range of problems, but they commonly occur in relation to teenagers and sexual health. Specific guidance (the Fraser guidelines) has been written for these areas; see 'Resources' at end of this appendix.

Autonomy and mental capacity

It is now generally accepted that patient autonomy is the overriding principle and should be respected above all others. But many GPs feel the same ethical tension between wanting to help our patients achieve autonomous goals whilst understanding that other patients, who may be less assertive, also need our time and care. We too are a rationed resource. To be truly autonomous one must obviously have the capacity to make decisions. This has always been implicitly understood but has now been made explicit by the *Mental Capacity Act* of 2005. (*The Mental Capacity Act* applies to England and Wales. Scotland has its own law, the *Scotland Mental Health Care and Treatment Act* of 2003 and in Northern Ireland *Common Law*, acting in patients' best interests, applies.)

> ### *Mental Capacity Act, 2005*
>
> Some of the provisions of the *Mental Capacity Act* are:
>
> Every adult must be assumed to have the capacity to make their own decisions unless proved otherwise (ie, do they have an impairment of brain or mind that makes them unable to understand and process the information?).
>
> Every 'capable' adult has the right to make what may be seen as unwise or eccentric decisions (eg, that branded Ventolin is better than salbutamol).
>
> Anything done on behalf of someone without capacity must be in their best interests and must be the option that is least restrictive to their personal liberty.

The *Mental Capacity Act* has important implications for GPs, particularly when we are assessing a patient's lack of capacity to make decisions and deciding how to act in a patient's best interests. For example, we may need to assess whether a patient has the **capacity** to **consent** to a proposed treatment. If they lack the capacity to do so, we must make a decision **in their best interests**. What these are cannot be assumed. Every effort should be made to enable their past feelings and values to be taken into account, and the views of those close to the person should also be considered.

Values-based practice

The traditional model of bioethics is very useful, but some argue that it may be too limited to help with the problems faced in modern practice. This is where values-based practice (VBP) can help. VBP is a framework that recognises that individual values and beliefs, both ours and those of our patients, will influence every healthcare encounter. But these values are often not elicited or recognised.

Your core belief, as well as the patient's, about whether or not Ventolin is better or not than generic salbutamol will obviously influence the outcome of your response to the above request. VBP is "an approach to link generalised scientific knowledge of evidence-based practice to the particular values of the patient" so that "the principles of evidence-based practice and values-based practice thus work together as a basis of shared decision making" (Petrova et al. *Br J Gen Pract* 2006;56:703–9). But there is also an ethical dimension because, as society becomes more heterogeneous, we no longer have the universal, shared values that have previously been taken for granted. A close examination of values suggests that the traditional model of bioethics has limitations. For example:

- Autonomy – while highly valued in Western societies as the overriding ethical priority, autonomy does not have a comparable value in more collectivist societies.

- Beneficence and nonmaleficence – the increasingly complex treatment options available to us mean that the application of these principles is not black and white. The simplest intervention (eg, an antibiotic for otitis media) may 'do good' for one person but 'do harm' for someone else. Evidence-based medicine is often criticised for being simplistic and reductionist but it has actually taught us that everything is more grey and complex. There are no absolutes, only relative benefits (numbers needed to treat) and relative harm (numbers needed to harm).

- Justice – as society becomes more heterogeneous, decisions regarding fairness and justice inevitably become more complex.

Ethical reasoning thus requires an exploration of differences in values rather than an attempt to define 'what is right'. VBP does not aim to provide knowledge about specific values, but to sensitise doctors to their own and their patients' values and the impact of these on decision making. The recognition of your own values is an important part of reaching out for the values of your patients and making shared decisions.

The GMC has produced guidance for doctors about religious and philosophical values (*Personal Beliefs and Medical Practice*, GMC, 2008). This acknowledges that doctors and patients have personal beliefs that are central to their lives and inevitably affect the consultation. We must treat our patients "with respect, whatever their life choices and beliefs", and take these values into account when making decisions. However, we must not allow any of our own personal beliefs or values to 'prejudice' our assessment of the patient's needs, or express these beliefs in a way that could cause them distress. If carrying out a certain procedure conflicts with your values (eg, referral for termination of pregnancy), you must explain this to the patient and tell them they have a right to see another doctor and make sure that they are able to do so.

Conclusion

Every day in general practice produces ethical dilemmas. These are complex, reflecting our heterogeneous postmodern society where nothing is certain and everything is relative. The traditional bioethical model (**autonomy, beneficence, nonmaleficence, justice, confidentiality** and **consent**) provides a useful framework for thought and reason, but we need to remember that individual values impact every decision. We must be sensitive to the particular values of our patients, ourselves and our colleagues.

Resources

General Medical Council. *Good Medical Practice.* London: General Medical Council, 2006. Available from: www.gmc-uk.org/guidance/good_medical_practice/GMC_GMP.pdf.

General Medical Council. *Personal Beliefs and Medical Practice.* London: General Medical Council, 2008. Available from: www.gmc-uk.org/guidance/ethical_guidance/personal_beliefs/ personal_beliefs.asp.

Royal College of General Practitioners. Curriculum Statement 3.3: Clinical Ethics and Values Based Practice. In: *Being a General Practitioner.* London: Royal College of General Practitioners, 2007.

Rogers W, Braunack-Mayer AJ. *Practical Ethics for General Practice.* Oxford: Oxford University Press, 2004.

Issues of consent and confidentiality for teenagers are common in the nMRCGP. For a useful guide to the ethical and legal principles see:

Larcher V. Consent, competence, and confidentiality. *BMJ* 2005:330:353–6.

For more on the implications of the *Mental Capacity Act* see:

Nicholson TR, Cutter W, Hotopf M, et al. Assessing Mental Capacity: The Mental Capacity Act. *BMJ* 2008;336:322–5.

Brown E, Pink J. Real life ethics: autonomy versus duty of care. *Br J Gen Pract* 2008;58:288–9.

Appendix 3:

Consultation models

According to the RCGP Curriculum, you must:

"[Demonstrate] familiarity with the common models of the consultation that have been proposed and how these models can be used to reflect on previous consultations in order to shape future consulting."

Curriculum for Specialty Training for General Practice. Being a General Practitioner. RCGP, 2007.

Why models?

If you haven't heard of consultation models before then we suggest you do a quick swot. The points below explain how they fit into normal practice. The table on page 105 gives you an at-a-glance guide, and the book list directs to you to more detail.

Models show and tell

Models are ways of looking at consultations in order to better understand and improve them. They are either:

- **task-orientated** – you need to do this, this and this (MRCGP, Pendleton et al., Stott and Davis, Neighbour; see the table)

- **descriptive** – when you watch doctors and patients, they do this, this and this (Tuckett et al., Byrne and Long; see the table)

- **explanatory** – this is why patients and doctors behave like this (Helman, Berne, Balint, Tuckett et al.; see the table)

Models help you to get somewhere

They can help you start the consultation, navigate it and end it.

Models give you the tools to become more skilled

'Nuff said.

Models give you frameworks

Models:

- make you safer (eg, 'safety-netting' from Neighbour's model)
- improve communication with the patient
- improve concordance
- improve doctor and patient satisfaction

Models are fun to play with

Soon you'll have finished the examination process and will start to enjoy yourself again. Consulting models are a good way to look afresh at your daily work, and to make your consultations better and better and better... Over the page is a table of our top 10 most relevant and important consultation models. Don't worry; you don't need to know them all! A passing knowledge of some of them, and why they are useful, will stand you in good stead. They may appear in the applied knowledge test, but we suggest that you discuss them with your trainer and agree on one or two with which to practise certain aspects of consulting. In reality, good consultations are influenced by bits of several different models, according to circumstance.

Ten important consultation models

Neighbour	Balint
Five consultation tasks are defined: 1. connecting 2. summarising 3. handing over 4. safety-netting 5. housekeeping	This is a psychotherapeutic approach. It involves a detailed analysis of the doctor–patient relationship. It promotes the idea of the doctor as a 'drug' – the most powerful therapeutic agent in the room. Balint case-discussion groups help the doctor to understand and cope with 'heartsink' patients.
Pendleton et al.	**Helman**
Seven consultation tasks are defined: 1. Define the reason for the patient's attendance (including the patient's ideas, concerns and expectations). 2. Consider other problems. 3. Choose an appropriate action for each problem. 4. Share understanding with the patient. 5. Involve the patient in the management plan. 6. Use time and resources well. 7. Establish and maintain a relationship with the patient.	Patients come to a consultation with six questions (folk model): 1. What happened? 2. Why did it happen? 3. Why me? 4. Why now? 5. What should I do about it? 6. What if I do nothing?
Tuckett et al.	**Berne**
The consultation is a meeting between experts: • Doctors are experts in medicine. • Patients are experts in their own illnesses. The aim is shared understanding, but: • Doctors rarely understand patients' beliefs. • And even more rarely address explanations in terms of the patient's belief system.	This is based on transactional analysis. Parent/adult/child roles are adopted by both the doctor and patient. The Berne model describes psychological games played by both the doctor and patient. It can be helpful with 'heartsink' patients.
Stott and Davis	**Calgary–Cambridge**
Four consultation tasks are defined: 1. management of presenting problems 2. management of ongoing heath problems 3. opportunistic health promotion 4. modification of health-seeking behaviours	This is a detailed descriptive guide to communication skills for the consultation. The use of silence at the start of a consultation to let the patient talk is encouraged.

Byrne and Long	Old MRCGP model (now used in COT)
Six phases to a consultation are defined: 1. The doctor establishes a relationship with the patient. 2. The doctor attempts to define the reason(s) for the patient's attendance. 3. The doctor examines the patient (verbal and/or physical). 4. The doctor (and patient) considers the problem(s). 5. The doctor (and patient) makes a management plan. 6. The consultation ends.	Discover the patient's reason for attendance: • Encourage that patient's contribution. • Respond to cues. • Place the complaint in a psychosocial context. • Explore the patient's health understanding. Define the clinical problem: • Include/exclude likely relevant significant conditions. • Make an appropriate physical/mental examination. • Make an appropriate working diagnosis. Explain the problem to the patient: • Use appropriate language and give an appropriate explanation. Address the patient's problem: • Seek to confirm the patient's understanding. • Provide an appropriate management plan. • Give the patient an opportunity to be involved in significant management decisions. Make effective use of the consultation: • Make effective use of resources/holistic care. • Ensure that the conditions and interval for follow-up are specified. • Check the patient's understanding of any medication prescribed.

Our two favourite models – a good place to start

Neighbour

Neighbour's model is (deceptively) simple, and very useful both in real life and for practising for the clinical skills assessment (CSA). It concentrates on good communication, sharing information and, unusually, on looking after yourself. It is based on good educational theory and analysis of communication skills. (And if you've read the book, you'll know that it's a bit offbeat too.) There are just five points to remember, one for each digit (unless you are a three-toed sloth, in which case you have probably fallen asleep before getting to this part of the book).

1. **Connect** – this is about listening skills, empathy and reaching shared understanding.

2. **Summarise** – this is about feeding back to the patient and checking understanding. Each time you are given a history try summarizing it – you'll be surprised at how effective this is!

3. **Handover** – this is about sharing the management plan and responsibility, ie, being patient-centred.

4. **Safety net** – this is about ensuring the patient knows when and why to come back, and remembering red flags. If you ensure that you 'safety net' in the CSA then you will gain marks.

5. **Housekeeping** – this is about reflecting, taking stock and looking after your own needs and health. In the CSA, this includes taking a drink of water and a deep breath, and clearing your mind for the next case.

Also, Neighbour talks about having two heads! Interested? Get the book!

Helman's model

Helman's model looks at the fascinating beliefs that people hold about why they get ill: it rained so I got flu, I ate too many chillies so my blood pressure went up, if I wrap myself up really warm my temperature will go down, my back aches so I must have a kidney infection... It's useful for considering why people present with complaints that, to doctors, might seem trivial, or present their complaints in ways that are hard to understand. Interested? Get this book too!

Resources

Essential guides

Tate P. *The Doctor's Communication Handbook*, 5th ed. Oxford: Radcliffe, 2006.

Thistlethwaite J, Morris P. *The Patient–Doctor Consultation in Primary Care: Theory and Practice*. London: Royal College of General Practitioners, 2007.

Original source publications

Balint M. *The Doctor, His Patient and the Illness*, 2nd ed. London: Churchill Livingstone, 2000.

Berne E. *Games People Play: the Psychology of Human Relationships*. London: Penguin Books Ltd, 1973.

Byrne PS, Long BE. *Doctors Talking to Patients*, revised ed. London: Royal College of General Practioners, 1984.

Helman CG. *Culture, Health and Illness*, 5th ed. London: Hodder Arnold, 2007.

Neighbour R. *The Inner Consultation: how to Develop an Effective and Intuitive Consulting Style*. Oxford: Radcliffe Medical Press, 2004.

Pendleton D, Schofield T, Tate P, et al. *The New Consultation: Developing Doctor–Patient Communication*, 2nd ed. Oxford: Oxford University Press, 2003.

Royal College of General Practitioners. *The General Practice Consultation*. London: Royal College of General Practioners, 2007. Available from: http://www.rcgp-curriculum.org.uk/ PDF/curr_2_The_GP_Consultation.pdf.

Silverman J, Kurtz S, Draper J. *Skills for Communicating with Patients*, 2nd ed. Oxford: Radcliffe Medical Press, 2004.

Stewart M, Roter D. *Communicating with Medical Patients*. Thousand Oaks, CA: SAGE Publications, 1989.

Stewart M, Brown JB, Weston WW, et al. *Patient-centred medicine transforming the clinical method*. 2nd edn. Abingdon: Radcliffe Medical Press; 2003.

Stott NC, Davis RH. The exceptional potential in each primary care consultation. *J R Coll Gen Pract* 1979;29:201–5.

Tuckett D, Boulton M, Olson C, et al. *Meetings Between Experts: an Approach to Sharing Ideas in Medical Consultations*. London: Routledge, 1985.

Usherwood T. *Understanding the Consultation: Evidence, Theory and Practice*. Buckingham: Open University Press, 1999.

Appendix 4:

Consultation observation tool marking schedule

Here is a blank version of the Expanded COT Marking Schedule for you to photocopy and use for practise.

Consultation observation tool guide				
Marking schedule	**Evidence**			
A. Discover the reason for patient attendance				
1. Encourages the patient's contribution • Attentive listening • Open questions • Nonverbal skills • Exploring and clarifying • Internal summaries • Signposting • Interruptions				
	Insufficient evidence	NFdev	Competent	Excellent
2. Responds to cues • Verbal • Nonverbal • Nonverbal response • Active response • Shows empathy				
	Insufficient evidence	NFdev	Competent	Excellent
3. Places complaint in psychosocial context • How problem affects patient/family • Patient's a				
	Insufficient evidence	NFdev	Competent	Excellent

4. Explores health understanding • Ideas, concerns, expectations • Curiosity • Discovers health beliefs				
	Insufficient evidence	NFdev	Competent	Excellent
B. Defines the clinical problem				
5. Includes or excludes likely relevant significant condition • Gathers information • Attentive listening • Open and closed questions • Appropriate questions • Internal summary/signposting • Pacing of questions • Use of existing knowledge/records • Medically safe				
	Insufficient evidence	NFdev	Competent	Excellent
6. Appropriate physical/mental examination • Choice of examination • Mental state examination • Examination explained in appropriate language • Sensitive approach • Targeted examination • Examination addresses patient's concerns				
	Insufficient evidence	NFdev	Competent	Excellent
7. Makes an appropriate working diagnosis • Integrates information • Recognises patterns of illness • Clinically sound hypothesis • Appropriate use of probability • Can analyse novel/unusual situations • Flexible use of rules and guidelines				
	Insufficient evidence	NFdev	Competent	Excellent

C. Explains the problem to the patient				
8. Uses appropriate language and give appropriate explanation • Patient centred • Use of patient's ideas and beliefs • Addresses concerns and expectations • Appropriate timing/pacing/language • 'Chunking' (ie, breaking the information down into manageable bits) and checking understanding • Internal summary/signposting • Varies explanatory techniques • Well organised and logical				
	Insufficient evidence	NFdev	Competent	Excellent
D. Addresses the patient's problem				
9. Seeks to confirm the patient's understanding • Actively confirms understanding of problem				
	Insufficient evidence	NFdev	Competent	Excellent
10. Appropriate management plan • Relates to working diagnosis • Good clinical practice • Appropriate investigations/referrals • Knows limits of competence • Shows knowledge of natural history of illness				
	Insufficient evidence	NFdev	Competent	Excellent
11. Patient is given opportunity to be involved in significant management decisions • Shares thoughts/involves patient • Negotiates • Offers choice/options • Encourages autonomy and opinions • Uses time as a therapeutic tool • Balanced plans, doctor/patient centred as appropriate • Evidence base used				
	Insufficient evidence	NFdev	Competent	Excellent

E. Makes effective use of the consultation				
12. Effective use of resources/holistic care • Understands socioeconomic /cultural background • Recognises doctor limitations • Uses of primary health care team and other resources • Use of complimentary medicine • Use of time				
	Insufficient evidence	NFdev	Competent	Excellent
13. Conditions and interval for follow up are specified • Safety netting • Timing appropriate • Confirm patient understanding				
	Insufficient evidence	NFdev	Competent	Excellent
14. Prescribing • Awareness of national and local guidelines • Checks understanding • Checks interactions/side effects • Cost effective • Can justify transgressions • Appropriate use of British National Formulary data				
	Insufficient evidence	NFdev	Competent	Excellent
Table courtesy of David Chidwick, Programme Director, Banbury Vocational Training Scheme. NFdev: needs further development.				

Index

A

AKT *see* applied knowledge test
ALLHAT *see* Antihypertensive and Lipid-Lowering
        Treatment to Prevent Heart Attack Trial
Anglo-Scandinavian Outcomes Trial (ASCOT) 30
Antihypertensive and Lipid-Lowering Treatment
        to Prevent Heart Attack Trial (ALLHAT) 30
applied knowledge test (AKT) 16, 32
    advantages of 17
    clinical questions, preparing for
        gap in knowledge and experience, identifying 19
        keeping cool, importance of 19–20
        keeping up to date 22–3
        major national guidelines, revision of 23
        MCQs, practising 23
        mind relaxation, importance of 24
        self-directed and needs-based learning strategy 20–2
    disadvantages of 18
    examination tips 30–1
    logistics of 18–19
    nonclinical questions, preparing for
        administration, management, ethics 24–5
        see also autonomy; bioethics;
            Mental Capacity Act; values-based practice
        research, EBM, CrAp, 25–6 *see also* CrAp/EBM,
    guide to question format
        data interpretation 29
        EMQ 26–7
        picture format 28
        seminal trials 29–30
        single best answer 26
        table/algorithm completion 27–8
    resources of 32–3
ASCOT *see* Anglo-Scandinavian Outcomes Trial
assessments
    clinical skills *see* clinical skills assessment (CSA)
    tools *see* consultation observation tool (COT)
    workplace-based *see* workplace-based assessment (WPBA)
autonomy, patient 100

B

bioethics 99, 101
    classic principles of 99
    limitations of 100
    usefulness of 99–100
BMJ Clinical Evidence guidelines 21
body language 49
'body talk' approach to consultation
    concept of 49, 54
    reasons for failure of 55
    tactics for ending consultation 54–5

C

'capturing' data 77
case-based discussion (CBD) 65
    concept of 67–8
    process of 68
    RCGP's question guide for 69–70
case–control studies 88
CBD *see* case-based discussion
CER *see* control event rate
certification, RCGP standard *see* RCGP Certification Unit
CIs *see* confidence intervals
clinical evaluation exercise *see* mini-clinical evaluation exercise
clinical management skills, explanation of 45
clinical questions, preparing for the AKT *see* applied knowledge test
clinical skills assessment (CSA) 35
    consulting skills, honing *see* consulting skills
    domain of 40
    dos and don'ts on day of 42–4
    golden rules for successful 41
    logistics of 37–8
    overview 36–7
    practising using marking schedule 44–6
    types of cases 38, 39
clinical supervisor's report (CSR) 65, 80
closed questions 49
cohort studies 88
communication skills 106

competency areas for assessment 10

concordance 47–8

Condensed Curriculum Guide, The 5

confidence intervals (CIs) 92–3

consultation models

    Balint 105

    Berne 105

    Byrne and Long 106

    benefits of 103–4

    Calgary–Cambridge 105

    Helman's model 105, 107

    Neighbour's model 105, 106–7

    old MRCGP model 106

    Pendleton et al. 105

    Stott and Davis 105

    Tuckett et al. 105

consultation observation tool (COT) 65

    assessor of 70

    desensitising exercises 71

    marking schedule, modified, of 73–7, 109–12

    process of 71

consulting room 37

consulting skills

    concordance 47–8

    consultation models 103–7

    cues, looking for 52–3 *see also* consultation observation tool

    ending consultations 53–5

    ideas, concerns, expectations 52

    list and agendas of patients 50, 51–2

    negotiating lists, tips for 51

    open questions 49

    patient-centredness 46–7

    starting consultations 48–9

control event rate (CER) 90, 91

COT *see* consultation observation tool

CrAp *see* critical appraisal

CrAp/EBM, guide to

    basic template for appraisal, making

        see evidence-based medicine

    definition and model 87

    PICO and 87–8

    sensitivity, specificity, predictive value, calculating 95–6

    statistical significance, assessing 92–3

    study types, understanding 88–9

    systematic reviews/meta-analyses, interpreting 94–5

    treatment effect, calculating 90–2

critical appraisal (CrAp)

    distribution of 17, 24

    preparation of 25

        see also CrAp/EBM, guide to

CSA *see* clinical skills assessment

CSR *see* clinical supervisor's report

D

data gathering, explanation of 45

deanery administrators 61

diagnostic studies

    calculating sensitivity and specificity in 95–6

    economic evaluations of 89

direct observation of procedural skills (DOPS) 65

    assessor of 79

    clinical skills assessed by 81–2

    concept of 79

    e-portfolio and 79, 81

    process of 79

disease-orientated evidence (DOE) 89

doctor–patient interaction *see* mini-clinical evaluation exercise

DOE *see* disease-orientated evidence

DOPS *see* direct observation of procedural skills

Duties of a Doctor Registered with the General Medical Council, The 3, 100

E

EBM *see* evidence-based medicine

economic evaluations 89

educational supervisor (ES) 59

    reviews 80

EER *see* experimental event rate

e-portfolio

    Clinical Encounter, recording 63

    concept of 61

    DOPS 79, 81–2

    guide to handling 64–5

    personal development plan, recording 63

    recording one's learning in 62–3

ES *see* educational supervisor

ethics 24, 58

    case-based discussion and 67

    dilemmas in 99

'e-ticket' 77

evidence-based medicine (EBM) 87–8

    basic template of

        allocation concealment 90

        intention-to-treat analysis 90

        relevance of study 89

        validity of study 89

    distribution of 17, 24

    preparation of 25

    see also CrAp/EBM, guide to

experimental event rate (EER) 90, 91

F

fitness 25, 58

G

General Medical Council (GMC) 2
    duties of doctors registered with 3
    Good Medical Practice, guidance of *see Good Medical Practice*
    guidance for doctors about religious and philosophical values
        see Personal Beliefs and Medical Practice
general practitioner (GP)
    clinical supervisor and 59
    community orientation work and 9
    comprehensive approach for patients 8
    core competencies needed in 7–9
    educational supervisor and 59
    e-portfolio 61–5
    general practice's application features 9–10
    GPT and 60
    MRCGP examination and 2 *see also* nMRCGP examination
    psychomotor skills 10
    RGCP curriculum for 6
    skills of, problem solving 7–8
    various roles of 11
GMC *see* General Medical Council
Good Medical Practice 3–4
GP *see* general practitioner
GPT *see* GP trainer
GP trainer (GPT) 60

H

Helman's model 105, 107

I

intention-to-treat analysis 90
interpersonal skills, explanation of 45
interpreting randomised controlled trials 29–30

K

key statements 12–13

L

learning
    needs-based 20–2
    recording *see* e-portfolio
    training-based 13, 58

M

MCQ *see* multiple choice question
Membership by module 12
Mental Capacity Act 100–1
meta-analysis 94–5
mini-CEX *see* mini-clinical evaluation exercise
mini-clinical evaluation exercise (mini-CEX) 65
    assessor of 72
    process of 72
    RCGP's definition of 71 *see also* consultation observation tool

Modernising Medical Careers programme 2
MRC-CUBE trial 30
MSF *see* multisource feedback
multiple choice question (MCQ) 16, 23, 32
multisource feedback (MSF) 65
    assessors 78
    concept of 77
    process of 78

N

National Institute for Health and Clinical Excellence (NICE) 21
negative predictive value (NPV) 95, 96
Neighbour's model 105, 106–7
NHS Clinical Knowledge Summaries 22
NICE *see* National Institute for Health and Clinical Excellence
nMRCGP examination
    AKT in *see* applied knowledge test
    CSA in *see* clinical skills assessment
    curriculum of 3–4 *see also* RCGP curriculum
    definition of 1–2, 3
    GMC's guidance 2
    'magic eye' pictures and 60
    mantra of 1
    relevance in real life 2–3
    Summative Assessment and 2, 13
    tips for enjoying 13
    working procedure of 12–13
    WPBA in *see* workplace-based assessment
NNT *see* number needed to treat
nonclinical questions, preparing for the AKT *see* applied
    knowledge test
NPV *see* negative predictive value
number needed to treat (NNT) 29–30, 90–2, 101

O

open questions 49

P

patient-centredness 46–7
patient-orientated evidence that matters (POEM) 89
patient satisfaction questionnaire (PSQ) 65
    assessors of 79
    explanation of 78–9
    process of 79
PDP *see* personal development plan
Personal Beliefs and Medical Practice 101
personal development plan (PDP) 63
person-centred care 7 *see also* patient-centredness
PMETB *see* Postgraduate Medical Education and Training Board
POEM *see* patient-orientated evidence that matters
positive predictive value (PPV) 95, 96
Postgraduate Medical Education and Training Board (PMETB) 2

PPV *see* positive predictive value
primary care management 7, 23–5
problem-solving skills 7–8
professionalism 58
professional values 58
PSQ *see* patient satisfaction questionnaire
P-value 92

Q

qualitative studies 89
question formats in the AKT *see* applied knowledge test

R

randomised controlled trials (RCTs) 88
    interpretation 29–30
RCGP Certification Unit 61
RCGP curriculum
    clinical skills, categorising 81–2
    contents of 6
    coping with 5–6
    core statement of
        essential application features 9–10
        psychomotor skills 10
        six core competencies 7–9
    domains derived from 40
    Good Medical Practice, based on 3–4
    nMRCGP competency areas and 10
RCTs *see* randomised controlled trials
'releasing' data 77

S

Scottish Intercollegiate Guidelines Network (SIGN) 21
sensitivity, diagnostic test 95–6
SIGN *see* Scottish Intercollegiate Guidelines Network
SnNout 96
specificity, diagnostic test 95–6
SpPin 96
statistical significance assessment
    CIs in 92–3
    P-value in 92
Summative Assessment 2, 13
systematic review 94–5

T

teamwork 58, 67, 70
TORCH *see* Towards a Revolution in Chronic Obstructive
             Pulmonary Disorder
Towards a Revolution in Chronic Obstructive Pulmonary
           Disorder (TORCH) 30
training 13–14
TRIP *see* Turning Research Into Practice
Turning Research Into Practice (TRIP) 22

V

values-based practice (VBP)
    approach of 101
    bioethics' limitations, identifying 101
    GMC's guidance on 101–2
VBP *see* values-based practice

W

WHI *see* Women's Health Initiative
Women's Health Initiative (WHI) 30
workplace-based assessment (WPBA) 16
    components of
        assessment of 68
        CBD 65, 67–70
        COT 65, 70–1, *see also* consultation observation tool
        CSR 65, 80
        DOPS 65, 79 *see also* direct observation
           of procedural skills
        educational supervisor's review 80
        mini-CEX 65, 71–7
        MSF 65, 77–8
        PSQ 65, 78–9
        timetable 67–7
        utility of 67
    concept of 58
    e-portfolio and 61–5
    handling failure of 84
    learning in hospital 83
    logistics of 59–60
    'magic eye' pictures and 60
    objective of 58
WPBA *see* workplace-based assessment

Special Offer for Revision Course Leaders and Postgraduate Tutors

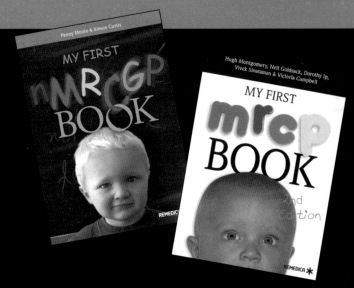

Remedica is delighted to provide significant discounts on bulk purchases of books for course students. For information and pricing on bulk purchases of *My First nMRCGP Book* and/or *My First MRCP Book Second Edition*, please contact:

Andrew Ward
Remedica Medical Education and Publishing
Commonwealth House
One New Oxford Street
London
WC1A 1NU
020 7759 2999
books@remedica.com

My First nMRCGP Book provides:

- a clear and logical explanation of the overall structure of the exam

- expert guidance on what trainees need to know for the exam and how to prepare for it

- an engaging, entertaining and educational read!

The second edition of *My First MRCP Book* now includes:

- fresh young authors

- new text to reflect the changes to the MRCP exam style

- the same juvenile sense of humour!